the WEIGH Way in

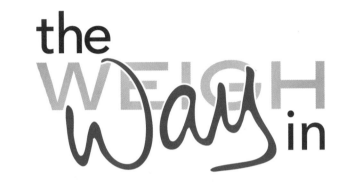

the Weigh in

5 Winning Strategies to Lose Weight, Get Strong and Lift Your Life

ANDREA MARCELLUS

AVROCK PRESS

The Way In
Copyright © 2019 Andrea Marcellus

ISBN: 978-1-7331518-2-5

Avrock Press
PO Box 56569
Sherman Oaks, CA 91413

FIRST EDITION

Designed by GKS Creative, Nashville

Illustrations by BrandXRepublic

Cover Photography by Timothy Norris
Additional Photography/Graphics by Isabel Rich

Library of Congress Control Number and PCIP on file with publisher

PRINTED IN CHINA

To my family and family of friends,

you lift my life and I love you dearly.

CONTENTS

1

I KNOW BECAUSE
I KNOW

OK, LET'S DO THIS. Here I am, your newly hired guide to fitness, eager to share all the wisdom I've earned through a quarter century of practical experience, my own insatiable curiosity and all the research I've done to answer questions and challenges posed by the hundreds of people whom I've had the privilege to guide.

But what I really want you to understand, right from the get-go, is that we are so in this together.

I know what you're feeling. I understand why you bought this book. I get what you're hoping to achieve and how frustrating it is to feel unable to attain your goals. Or to get to a "goal weight" and then not be able to stay there.

And the reason I understand all of this is because I've been through it. And around it. And on top of it. And underneath it. I know what you feel because *I know*.

Unlike most of the amazing trainers I've met, I was never a gifted athlete. In fact, the only athletic thing I ever did right in my entire life was by accident. In eighth grade, I tried out for field hockey at a new school and barely made the team.

I rarely got to play. But during the last game of the season, the coach finally put me in. It was a genuinely nauseating moment, but also a thrilling opportunity. I rushed onto the field determined to make a difference and, as fate would have it, within twenty seconds I managed to score the only goal of the game! What?! Me? Yes! Was it my talent?

Not exactly. The only reason I scored was because a defender hit the ball and it bounced off my stick as I happened to be standing in front of the goal. Also, in the spirit of full disclosure, I should mention that I, too, was a defender, which means I was on the wrong side of the field. I wasn't exactly the MVP.

Similarly, unlike many of my super-awesome Pilates colleagues, I was never a very good dancer. This fact was cemented after my first musical audition at NYU. Acting, singing and dancing had been my life since I was three, so I was shocked when parts were announced, and I didn't even get a role in the chorus, let alone the leading role I coveted. Still, there was hope: The Assistant Director—a friend of my roommate—sent her home with a personal message for me. (I mean, why would he bother? I hadn't even gotten cast!) But then it occurred to me: *OMG, he sought me out. Could it be he thinks so much of my overall talent that he wants to help me?* As it turned out, he did!

Sort of. What the Assistant Director wanted me to know was that my acting was strong, and so were the 16 bars I sang. His advice was this: Do not ruin those things by trying to dance. Certainly not as a professional. Maybe not even drunk at a wedding.

Considering that I'm a highly coordinated person, you can imagine how surprised I was by the newsflash that I was the comic relief at a dance audition. But don't be sad for me. This feedback, though harsh, turned out to be a great act of kindness. I swallowed my pride, decided I don't have to be good at everything and refocused my energy on the skills that would allow me to stand out. And after that, I went on to win many leading roles — all of them suited for the (I still take issue with this) "rhythmically-challenged."

Lastly, in the realm of things I am not (and the most relevant to you, dear reader), I was never a skinny-minnie. I was always healthy and "fine." But even in my early 20's, when I was teaching between 8 and 15 fitness classes each week, weight-lifting on my own time before and after my full-time executive assistant job, and literally running to and from acting auditions in whatever minutes I could squeeze between work and nightly play rehearsals, I was never super-lean. And believe me, I was motivated. I did it "right."

As you probably know, competition for professional acting roles is fierce. And believe it or not, I was always kind of the "big" girl in the room.

When you spend half of your days in commercial audition waiting rooms, looking around at 30 women who look like bizarro-clones of you, you become acutely aware of your "type." There are the women who do luxury-car and beer commercials, and women who sell potato chips and spray cleaner. We all want to be a luxury-car lady. A beer beauty. But me? It became apparent very quickly that I belonged in the domain of spray cleaners. Not just spray cleaners, of course; sometimes I was a mustard mom, or a Kmart shopper, or a woman who frequents some bank I can't remember. But the point remains: I had a spray-cleaner body in a beer-worshipping world.

Regardless, my confidence had been set in stone by a multitude of leading roles I had won in small-scale New York theaters and low-budget indie films. I honestly believed I stood a great chance at turning my skills into a lucrative career. I just had to make some changes. And since the best opportunities and more prominent parts seem to go to the genetically blessed, I knew what I needed to do: anything and everything I could to be "more." And that didn't just mean working harder and being more dedicated. Being more meant weighing less.

Believing that size was the lynchpin to my success as both an actress and a fitness instructor, I followed conventional wisdom to a tee, working out harder and eating "better" (meaning more and more restrictively) as I tried to become leaner, fitter, and more than just "regular." But despite years of researching and testing every workout and eating plan that made sense, I never found the holy grail that would make me super-lean. I did get fitter. I did look better. But I definitely didn't *feel* better.

Hyper-attention to my body left me just as critical of myself, if not more. Physically, I was still nowhere close to what I thought I would look like after working out that hard, for that long, all while being that "good" with my eating. I know many of you feel my pain on that point.

It's crucial to understand that my failure to achieve some sort of uber-fit-looking body was mainly because my goals themselves were misguided. The relentless focus on perfecting what I thought the world wanted to see on my outside, rather than valuing the unique skills and abilities I had inside, left me feeling constantly defeated. Without even realizing it, I was operating from a place of perceived "lack" and discounting my strengths. Let's think about this for a second: no matter your talents and gifts, how far can you really get in life if you tell yourself every day that you aren't good enough? In my case, the answer was not very far. Those years were grueling, exhausting, soul-stripping, and stressful. So, so, so stressful.

But never fear, we're not here to rehash my past insecurities—that's what my "ladies' night out" is for. The point is that I totally get why you bought this book. I get that, while we all agree that health is important, you are probably motivated to "diet" and "get fit" because you are unhappy with the way you look. You want—and maybe need—a big change, and I take great pride in helping people achieve bodies they never thought possible. But we can't do it by hating on ourselves. The only way you'll succeed is by shifting your attention away from perceived shortcomings to newly created habits and to-do's that improve not just your appearance and health, but your life as a whole.

The goal of this book is to have you adopt, step by step, The Way In lifestyle. Ending up with a fitter, leaner body will undoubtedly be a result—but it's not the most important one, and it can't be the primary focus.

It is crucial to look at the big picture, not just the mirror.

Your most significant achievement when you implement this plan will be mastering your own mind. The body of your dreams (and just about anything else you can dream up) will become far more possible as a result.

During the first 16 years of my fitness career, I became a knowledgeable, respected professional with a stable business and a devoted following. But while I was doing my best to be an inspiring mentor and improve the health of my clients, I knew something was missing. I knew in my heart I could only help people get to a certain level. And I knew this because, despite doing everything I was "supposed" to, I could only get *myself* to a certain level. That dissatisfying truth gnawed away at me until finally, one day, I decided to privately and quietly offer myself up as a guinea pig for my own terrifying experiment: I would do *less*. (Shudder!)

In fact, I would do basically the *opposite* of everything I had been doing in my career up to that point. Every day, I would do exactly what *felt* right, rather than what I was "supposed" to do. I did resistance workouts (anything using gym equipment, Pilates machines, weights, bands, balls, etc.) for only 20 minutes at a time and only a few days a week—a massive change for someone who had worked out hard three or four times per week (on top of cardio) for 18 years. Instead of hard interval cardio or running, I would walk or do a moderate session on a piece of cardio equipment every single day—but again only for 20-30 minutes at a stretch. Instead of working out so much, I would simply stand and move around each day as much as possible.

The other, even scarier part of the plan had to do with food. Not only would I work out less, I would also eat more. Not in terms of portion, but in terms of *kind*. I would ratchet down the size of my meals, but I wouldn't worry so much about *which* foods I ate. Instead, I would think about food being for energy and schedule and portion my meals accordingly. This meant, a few times a week, I would skip the judgment and let myself have the pizza. When my husband and I had guests for Sunday dinner, I'd ignore the giant bowl of steamed veggies and say, "pass the rigatoni." Out with the frozen yogurt and in with the real ice cream. Out with the protein bars and in with the nut-butter sandwich on whole-wheat bread (gasp!). I would say "yes, please" more than "no, thank you."

And I shrunk.

The Plan Makes The Body, The Mentality Makes It Permanent

Even more importantly, I started to smile again. Like, for real. I mean, I always wore a big smile, and it wasn't disingenuous. I love life, and I'm always excited to see what adventures the day will bring. But, like many world-class perma-smilers, my brightness and optimism during my 20's and early 30's was sometimes just a habit. A choice I made. A daily ritual to guard against the darkness in my life, both circumstantial and self-inflicted. Your new guide, like many of you, is a survivor of some unfortunate circumstances, crushing disappointments, and steep consequences for her own horrible choices. Smiling through stuff has always been my way. But when I stopped policing myself, and when I started to live with more freedom, I stopped smiling by rote. Now when I smile, it comes from deep confidence and the peace of knowing I can attain even the most elusive of personal goals.

Focusing on a personally authentic, intuitive approach to fitness not only got me the lean, strong, flexible body I always wanted, it also helped me develop a healthier, far more appreciative mentality. I gained new clarity in my life and re-discovered the kind of self-assurance we all start with as children but seem to lose somewhere along the way. There's a precious time in our lives when the world is still just a big, curious place full of opportunity. A time when we never question whether or not we can accomplish things—we just dream them up and assume it'll work out. A time when we feel complete "as-is," not waiting for some imaginary greatness that will come "when X happens," or if "I can manage to do Y," or "if I could just look like _____." I began to honestly believe so deeply and unshakably something I hadn't since I was a kid: I already have everything I need in my head and my heart to make extraordinary things happen. That I am, and have always been, enough.

The Way In is how I uncovered my best self yet. And that's exactly what I want for you.

2

YOUR BEST BODY
IS ALL IN YOUR HEAD

FULL DISCLOSURE: This is exactly the kind of chapter I would totally blow through. If you are anything like my type-A self, you are thinking, *"OMG. Skip the touchy-feely stuff. Just tell me what to do, and I'm on it."* I like rules, parameters. Give me a guide, a diagram, three easy rules and I'm set. Even better if I start to see results, right?

But there's a reason your açai-syrup-paprika-water-kombucha-cleanse gave you both immediate weight loss and long-term disappointment. I can give you the rules for a diet that will help you fit into a smaller size of jeans—and it would be a sane diet that won't require you to give up solid foods or turn you into a raging hunger-fueled crab-monster. But even a healthy, sustainable diet without the right mindset is going to let you down at some point. I've seen it over and over again in my clients, and yes, in myself. It's like buying a cheap eyebrow pencil—it might look good on you for a little while, but as soon as the going gets tough and you start to sweat, suddenly your perfectly shaped brows look like you melted a brown crayon on your forehead. So, stick with me here. Because I promise you, your best body starts with your best brain.

Killing Ourselves to Weigh-In

In 2005, the founder of CrossFit was interviewed by the New York Times about whether or not the exercise regimen was too extreme to be healthy. After all, devotees of the gym franchise can be found conquering daunting Olympic ™ gymnastics rings, running military-style drills, and even carrying gigantic logs. In CrossFit circles, people will beam with pride as they tell you harrowing tales of collapsing during workouts or throwing up from exhaustion. The founder's response to this criticism? "It can kill you. I've always been completely honest about that." And given the number of injuries that CrossFit has produced as it becomes one of the fastest growing fitness trends in the world, he might just be right.

I'm going to go out on a limb here and guess that you, reader, don't feel like killing yourself—literally or figuratively—for a workout trend. You are most likely not a professional athlete. You're probably not training to go to war. And you're certainly not a lumberjack. So why exercise like one?

"Fitness," it seems, has become synonymous with pain and punishment. And the way we approach nutrition is often no different. From fasting to diets that eliminate not just one food group but *half the pyramid*, we're often told that the only way to live a healthy life is to get rid of all the foods that make it worth living. Fat is bad, and sugar is bad, and gluten is bad, and most of all, *we* are bad if we eat them. Every meal we eat comes with a side of shame and guilt.

Weigh-in after weigh-in, we look to a number on a scale to tell us if we're enough, if we're worthy, if we finally deserve to be happy. And when the diet fads and fitness crazes are over, we still find ourselves locked out of the life we want—without any idea of how to get in.

That's what this book is about: *A better way in.*

It starts with letting go of all the shame and guilt and the punishment mentality you've been holding on to for so long and reimagining what life could be like without them.

I know, I know, it's easier said than done. If you're a woman, there's a good chance you've hated the way you look for almost as long as you were tall enough to see yourself in the bathroom mirror. But that's why we're here.

Over the years, training athletes, celebrities, and housewives alike; navigating the cutthroat entertainment industry and generally learning to turn a whole bunch of lemons into lemonade, I've developed a code to help me and the people I work with get their minds in shape. I've created what I call the "5 Life Strategies" to help you lay an all-new foundation of confidence and self-reliance. And while they are a critical part of losing weight and getting physically healthier, they're also tools you can use to set any goal and stay on a path to achieving it.

> **THE 5 LIFE STRATEGIES**
>
> ❗ **Practice Personal Authenticity**
>
> ⚙ **Strategize Habits**
>
> ★ **Live The Rule Of Awesome**
>
> ☯ **Develop Oppositional Stability**
>
> ✺ **Allow In The Extraordinary**

The Way In will not only leave you a better version of yourself, but more importantly, you'll also finish with the skills you need to maintain any goal and keep going. And as you do, you'll change your life in a way no amount of weight loss ever could.

Got that? Yes, you're going to lose weight. Yes, you're going to feel healthier. But unlike that cheap eyebrow pencil, when the going gets tough, you're not going to become a mess. You're not going to descend into a puddle of shame-spiraling or guilt-racked binges. The 5 Life Strategies will help you feel more in control of your life, more able to adjust to difficult circumstances, and to actually like what you see in the mirror—no matter what the scale says.

Practice Personal Authenticity—Be the best you, not someone else

It's time to get real with yourself. Not "social media real." Not "drunken confessional real." Really real. Who are you? What do you like? What are your stumbling blocks? And just as importantly, what are all the great, amazing, unique things that make you *you*.

Getting more out of life means being honest with yourself about your strengths and weaknesses. That's the only way you can improve those areas you're not happy with and learn to use all of your talents and skills unapologetically and to your greatest advantage.

But personal authenticity isn't just about who you are... it's also about who you're not. We all occasionally look at people in our lives, or on the pages of a magazine, and wish we were more like them. A lot of the time, that person you see is a carefully curated illusion created by amazing photoshop skills or Instagram filters (and yes, she probably did *buy* all those cupcakes for the bake sale, OK?).

But even if it's not an illusion, other people can't be our goals. When we let ourselves get wrapped up in impossible role models or other peoples' expectations, we can't help but focus on our supposed "lack"—our "shortcomings." Of course, we all want to improve who we are, and we should! No one is perfect, and we should strive to become better versions of ourselves. But that's the key: better versions of *us*, not someone else. True freedom comes from creating positive parameters through self-knowledge and then honoring them. Creating this space for yourself, to embrace who you are—the good, the bad, and the brilliant—will give you the motivation and road map to power your life forward.

Strategize Habits
—Be a little thoughtless

If you're anything like me, every single day, you are asked to make somewhere between three and 3 million decisions. Every one of those decisions takes up your time and makes that next decision a little bit more difficult. Psychologists call this "decision fatigue," and it's been theorized that this is the reason Steve Jobs wore the same thing every day, as do others of the ilk.

If we can get rid of some of those extraneous decisions, we can de-stress our lives and free up mental space for the choices that really matter. In a way, strategizing your habits is the opposite of the last rule. If it doesn't matter, make it easy. Think ahead for things like meals you eat alone every day or morning workout routines. Have go-to outfits and nightly habits that get you the sleep you know you need. If you create a strategy for the not-so-consequential tasks, you'll begin to do the smart, healthy, easy thing by rote, freeing up your brain for more important, exciting and fulfilling things.

THE WAY IN TO SUCCESS:
Name It and Claim It

Journeys of change are so often motivated by a feeling of "lack"—lacking what others have, lacking the qualities of the person you desire to become, lacking the life you want. But this perception of lack can set us up for failure—especially in the long term.

There will always be times when what we don't have is an important motivator. But when life throws us curveballs—whether it's a sugar-filled day at the carnival, flirting with ill-advised bangs, or a passive-aggressive call from your sister—we need something to run towards, not away from, and a number on the scale just isn't going to cut it.

Yes, I'm talking about life goals. Purpose. Direction. Who you want to be and what you want to offer out to the world?

It's OK to feel freaked out. Admitting to what we want is actually one of the hardest things. And putting it down on paper makes it even more dauntingly real. But I'm not letting you off the hook—this is too important. Right now, this second, write down the answers to these questions:

Life List

- *List 3-5 big things you would do this year if money and time were no issue.*

- *List 3-5 things you can accomplish in 20 minutes. (Yes, even those things - ha!)*

- *List three subjects you wish you knew more about.*

- *List three things you can do but wish you were better at.*

CONGRATULATIONS! You now have a list of go-to life-elevating "to-do's" for times when you would normally turn to food to soothe yourself or try to fill some of the holes we all have in our lives.

Laminate your Life List and keep it in your desk and in the cupholder in your car and on the top shelf of the fridge and taped to the bathroom mirror. It won't refocus your nervous or sad energy every time. But if it even works 25% of the time, you'll be on your way toward a more enriched (and leaner) life! Plus, now you're clearer about the possibilities before you. Make the realm of possibility your favorite mental vacation destination - the perception of lack can't exist there!

LIFE LIST

STRIVE AND THRIVE: big things you would do this year if money and time were no issue

_____

_____

_____

_____

_____

SEE SUCCESS: things you need to do that get back-burnered, and that can be accomplished in 20 minutes

_____

_____

_____

_____

_____

CULTIVATE CURIOSITY: subjects you wish you knew more about

_____

_____

_____

CREATE CONFIDENCE: skills you have but wish you were better at

_____

_____

_____

**Live the Rule of Awesome—Just say "no"
...or "yes!"**

This might be the easiest rule to remember, if not to execute. It's very simple: If it's not awesome, don't do it.

OK, OK, sometimes you have to do things that aren't awesome, especially if we're talking about changing diapers or helping with Algebra homework. Please don't use me as an excuse to make your spouse do all the dishes. Some things in life, despite their distinct un-awesomeness, must be done.

But for a lot of things—more things than we are often willing to admit—we do have a choice. That candle party you don't want to go to, but you feel bad, and you're gonna spend the entire 3 hours watching the clock and eating bland appetizers because you're bored out of your mind, and you don't even want candles anyway? Yeah, that's not awesome. And you really don't have to do it. That sweater you splurged on, but doesn't fit you right and makes you feel like a link sausage? Get rid of it. The too-saucy pizza you don't even like? Don't eat it. If the choice in front of you doesn't bring you joy and make you feel fabulous, choose something else.

Now, if it is awesome? Do it! Have the dammed piece of cake! Go out dancing! Buy yourself those shoes—your legs look amazing in them. The point is if you're going to make a choice, make one with clarity and purpose. Think of the last time you were at a buffet. Chances are, you ate a ton of food that was absolutely terrible for your health, and you didn't even enjoy it. Some splurges, some extravagances, some distractions are worth it. And some really aren't. The Rule of Awesome is about knowing the difference. Life's too short to waste time, energy and calories on things that don't make you happy.

 **Embrace Oppositional Stability
—Bend so you don't break**

In Pilates, there's a concept that says if your body needs to bend in one direction, energy must first initiate in the opposite direction. In other words, when you want to bend left, first move right to give yourself balance and a solid base from which to move. Think about being pushed by someone much stronger than yourself. If you try to stand straight and rigid, you'll

THE WAY IN TO SUCCESS:
Curiosity Rather than Judgment

Remember when you were a kid, and the world was full of possibility? Everywhere around you were questions, and you were excited to explore every single one.

Adults, however, tend to see the world in terms of answers. We know everything, especially when it comes to ourselves, and most likely, we've got a basket full of judgments to accompany every "fact" we know.

The Way In asks you to rediscover curiosity about yourself and the magic of "what if..."

> ***What if:***   *you didn't change a single food you eat, but simply adjusted your portioning method?*
>
> ***What if:***   *you stood an extra 60 minutes every day this week?*
>
> ***What if:***   *you experimented to see how and if certain foods affect your body?*

Each week, I'm going to ask you to find out something new about yourself—the rules of your own body and how it works best. Rather than judging who you are, what you're capable of, and what you think you know, come to this process with curiosity. Let's find out, together, what you like, what you don't like, which foods and exercises and routines help you feel and look your best. Let's find out what "The Rule of Awesome" means to you.

fall over. If you absorb the energy and move backward, you're able to keep your balance and then move forward again.

Life is continually trying to push us over. From fights with your spouse to parenting challenges, to that vacation you're not sure if you can afford, to that boss who thinks taking care of your sick kid is a vacation day—when we get hit, we often want to run, shut down and become immobile, or look for something heavy to throw at the offending party (just kidding).

But instead of those unhelpful impulses, there's a fourth option: absorb the hit and step in the opposite direction before you respond. Consider the other person's point of view and their motivations first. And while you are doing that, your anger, hurt or frustration has a moment to dissipate. You can tap into your empathy and rationality, which gives you a better base from which to respond. And after you consider your husband's complaint, your child's excuse, or Jeff's workaholic point-of-view, you might still be absolutely right. But your new perspective will help you formulate a response that is balanced, fair, and ultimately, more effective.

 ## Allow in the Extraordinary—Take a detour to greatness

How many times have you thought, "if I could just get/do/have X, my life would be so much better?" If you're reading this book, you've probably thought that about a number on the scale. But maybe it's a new house, a prettier wardrobe, a better job. Perhaps it's a husband or wife. We're all on a journey to get somewhere, and it's tempting to put our hands on the steering wheel and lock our eyes on that horizon. Take it from someone who drives in Los Angeles, you may get there eventually, but is sitting in traffic for half your life the best way to spend your time?

"The Rule of Awesome" is about discernment —about making the choice that makes you feel awesome. But "Allow in the Extraordinary" is about permission. I'm giving you permission to go out there and find things that bring you joy. Get out of the car! Take the detour! Breathe in the sweet summer air and stretch your legs! Too often we find ourselves waiting around for something incredible to happen to us. But even diamonds don't shine unless you take the time to cut and polish them. We have to seek out those moments that make life worth living. The road to extraordinary isn't a straight trip. It's a stolen mile every day.

One More Thing

These 5 Life Strategies will be a foundation of the work we're going to do together. Because The Way In isn't a diet; it's a lifestyle. And just like any life endeavor, your mentality is the most significant component of your success or failure. It might sound new-agey, but you will not achieve permanent results without finding a way to actively love and appreciate my new favorite client: you!

I can almost hear you thinking, *If you're going to tell me to look in the mirror, wrap my arms around myself and say something like "Someone special deserves a hug!" I'm not doing it.*

Please. I already admitted I'm totally type-A and, honestly, the only time I stop to actively appreciate myself in some touchy-feely way is when I go to meditation class where I'm forced to be quiet and breathe and then the instructor says something about being a warrior against life's hardships and a champion who endures by putting one foot in front of the other no matter what's in the way... and tears start pouring out every time.

But I digress. And I'm not interested in motivational slogans – you've already got Pinterest for that. I'm all about practical strategies for adjusting your mentality to get you to your goals faster. And we're starting with what you see when you look in the mirror. So, brace yourself, go to a mirror and take a good look.

Really?

Yes, really.

Now?

Yes. Bring the book with you.

Mirror, mirror on the wall...who's the meanest one of all? (The answer is probably YOU.)

When you look in the mirror, are you looking for what's right or to check out what's wrong? Think about it the next time you look. What strikes you first: something about you that rocks, or something that you'd like to hide from the world?

For many of us, conversations with the mirror go something like this:

BAD DAY CONVERSATIONS: *Seriously?! How did my ass get bigger over-night? It was only one piece of bread at dinner!!...OK, that's it. I'm never eating out again...Except for when I don't feel like cooking...which is multiple nights a week...OK screw it. I'm just going to get bigger pants.*

GOOD DAY CONVERSATIONS: *Ok, somehow my ass doesn't look SO bad in these pants. Guess I'll wear them, but I'll definitely do the long sweater or shirt I can tie around my waist just in case.*

RARE TO NEVER CONVERSATIONS: *Hey, there good-looking! Look at you. You're awesome. And you're me! So, I guess that's working out pretty well for us!*

The trouble for many of us when we look in the mirror is, we don't know who we're looking for. It's as if the person we see there is someone we don't particularly like but have to put up with. It's jarring to think of ourselves—and our bodies—as a nuisance that we can't get rid of. It's also incredibly de-motivating. What's the use of trying to be our best selves if we always come back to "not good enough?" The ironic truth is that too much focus on your body often gets in the way of improving it.

Your weight loss journey affects your exterior, for sure. But the best results are not achieved by focusing on what other people see. Better Instagram selfies aren't motivation enough to change your life in a deep and meaningful way. Instead, we are going to work on **uncovering** your best self which, believe me, is already there.

IF *THE WAY IN* IS ABOUT ANYTHING,

IT'S ABOUT, FINALLY AND FOREVER, ONCE AND FOR ALL,

GETTING YOUR OUTSIDE TO MATCH THE PERSON

YOU KNOW YOU ARE ON THE INSIDE.

In order to do that, we have to rethink the mirror. So, for the next 6 weeks, rather than using the mirror to make judgments about your appearance, let's just use it as a place to check-in. A sort of sounding board to help you make decisions about **what you are going to DO with your time**. I mean, yes, you can also use it to make sure you didn't misalign your buttons. But then it's practice time:

MAKING THE MIRROR A USEFUL TOOL:
Eight Breaths to a Better Mood

MIRROR MOOD-LIFTER ONE: GRACE

Take a breath (yes, literally do this) and look. Hold the air inside your lungs until you find one "thumbs up" thing about what you see. As you exhale, let go of everything else except that one acceptable (if not totally fabulous) thing. Mentally zeroing in on this one thing, take two more breaths, and with each exhale, allow yourself to more deeply appreciate your "thing."

Please don't think I'm suggesting you make googly-eyes at yourself in the mirror or start chanting. Just look... accept... and allow some grace to exist in your heart for yourself.

(BTW... if you turn purple and fall over, this is 100% a sign you are way too hard on yourself. Just the fact that you have access to this book means something is going right in your life. Try again and maybe focus on that.)

MIRROR MOOD-LIFTER TWO: ACTION

Take a breath (yep, it's still all about the breathing) and think of your Life List. Keep your breath still until you choose one item on your list to give your exhale. Do this two more times, allowing the probability of accomplishing the item to grow:

Exhale acceptance that the person in the mirror CAN accomplish the Life List item. It doesn't mean you will or that you must – the key is telling yourself that, if you choose, if you put your mind to it, you can.

On the next breath, hold it still until you pick one step you can easily do to move toward that goal. Giving yourself one step of the HOW you will accomplish your goal, solidifies the CAN.

On the last breath, allow your mind to say when. Go with whatever first pops into your head... be it, next week, or now or two months from now. Like reading a novel, picking a date helps create the story – a mental picture immediately appears of you accomplishing the goal in a particular place, during a season and at a certain time of day, with this person or that person... you get the idea. The clearer and more detailed that picture becomes over time, the more likely you are to keep that date with yourself.

See? No self-hugs here. I'm not asking you to *artificially appreciate* the person you are. A forced, inauthentic moment is not going to help. But seeing yourself, with love and honesty will help you put that mirror to good use. Use the moment to refocus negative mental energy toward your Life List and allow that to be energized instead of your self-doubt.

Eventually, you'll go from seeing the things that are OK, to realizing you're flat-out fabulous.

Seriously?

Yes.

Change is all about breaking patterns, including our mental patterns about ourselves. We need to replace the tired song of woe we play endlessly in our heads with new music that stirs up energy and purpose. The way to do that isn't by talking about what we've done wrong, or what we want to do, but by thinking up positive steps, even small ones, and taking them. As you make commitments to do something every day, bit by bit, you'll start to impress yourself. Your mind will begin to calm, and your heart will heal. It just happens.

After a while, when you look in the mirror, the first thing you see won't be what's wrong. It'll be a person you've been getting to know who does so much right. A capable person who, just like every other human, has a few things that could use improvement... but overall has a leg up in life simply for being able to shift mental woe into mental "let's go."

Remember? No more pain and punishment. No more killing ourselves "death by 1000 cuts-style" every time we go to the gym, or open a magazine or watch a TV show. No need to tear yourself down to build yourself back up. Nope. Not you. Starting right where you are at, we will begin by building off of what is going right in your life. Your mind is calm. Your heart is open, and your head is protected by a hard hat of goals and solid direction. We're building something here, and that thing is a better you.

3

SETTING YOURSELF UP
TO SUCCEED

I'M GOING TO LET YOU IN ON A LITTLE SECRET I've learned after years of training people from all walks of life: There's no such thing as an average person.

Well, now, that's statistically impossible, you may be thinking. But that's just it. Statisticians may find averages and means useful, but for real, living people, they don't mean much.

The best example I can give to illustrate my point is caloric recommendations. How many calories should you eat each day? That's easy! The answer is 2,000, and we know that because the FDA tells us so. But where does that number come from?

In 1993, the year I started teaching fitness classes, the FDA decided to make recommendations on caloric needs based on findings by the National Academy of Science. In the midst of a growing obesity crisis, it seemed a logical step to help people understand nutrition. Armed with studies and statistics, it settled on one nice, round number to apply to the "average" American: 2,000. Easy peasy. And with this new 2,000 calorie guide, Americans could design a healthy daily plan by simply looking at the side of a food package and doing some basic math.

The problem is that the number of calories you *need* in a day is related to the number of calories you *burn* in a day, and that is dependent on a number of factors. How old are you? Are you male or female? How tall are you? Are you drinking enough water? Are you active? Are you particularly stressed? Are you getting enough sleep? Are your in-laws visiting? Are you on vacation? OK, those last two may not be relevant, but you get the point. Even an "average" height, "average" weight, "averagely" active person may still need more or less than 2,000 calories. They could need more when they work at a hotel front desk, standing all day, and less when they get a new job where they sit.

This isn't a slam on the FDA—they are trying to be helpful, after all. But it comes down to this: *food labels are NOT meant to be a prescription for what you "should" be doing.* The 2,000 calorie "ideal" may not apply to you at all. In my opinion (and since you bought this book, I assume you're asking), it most likely doesn't. After 25 years of helping clients achieve fitness goals and watching our lives become increasingly more sedentary, 2,000 calories is **way too much** for most women and, yes, many men as well.

The bottom line is that diet rules made by someone who doesn't know your body can only go so far. You have strengths and weaknesses, and a million fantastic quirks. You have different energy needs than me, or your coworkers, or even your twin sister. You have different needs from day to day.

That's why (to say it again) The Way In is a lifestyle—guided by me, but designed by *you,* for *your* body.

Some of you are reading this and thinking, *Yes! I want a plan that's based on listening to my own needs!*

Some of you are thinking: *Can't you just give me a formula? Preferably something I can enter into a slick app on my phone?*

I have good news and bad news for you: Yes, there is an app that can help (my AND/life app). No, it's not going to give you a chart of your measurables and make math out of your fitness journey.

I get it, numbers make us feel like we're in control. The fitness industry is booming right now with apps and calculators and gizmos and gadgets, all to help us monitor the calories we theoretically take in and the energy we supposedly put out. But if all this technology—the "metric-ization" of our health, as I call it—is really helping, why are so many of us still struggling to reach our fitness goals? It's because while numbers don't lie, they don't tell the whole story either. The simple calories-in/calories-out approach leaves an essential piece out of the equation: *You are not a machine.*

When you put your hope in a watch or your place on a chart, there's a flip side as well: the strong disappointment you feel when you fail to live up to your numerical expectation. Even worse is when your numbers all add up but, somehow, your scale doesn't reflect that. It's one more way we equate food and activity—and by extension ourselves as people—with "good" and "bad."

You are an individual; you are not average, and your fitness program shouldn't be either.

In the next chapter, I'm going to give you the specific guidelines you'll need to begin designing your own "way in." But before we get there, I want you to understand the big ideas these guidelines are based on.

Extremism is Destructive

Calorie *awareness* is a far better technique to employ than calorie *counting,* especially since there's no point in measuring your intake based on height/ weight averages of other people. The Way In uses a no-brainer, visual portioning method so you'll never need a measuring cup or calculator to have lunch. This method will teach your stomach to crave smaller amounts of food over time, so while you aren't counting calories, you will be eating fewer of them. And unlike arbitrary diet rules based on measuring or tracking, you'll stop eating because it *feels* right, not out of guilt or obligation. A lifestyle where you feel restricted is simply unsustainable. You will inevitably yo-yo between being hungry or grumpy or unsatisfied, aka, "good," and being carefree and indulgent, aka, "bad."

By following your body instincts, you'll develop a more authentic and pleasurable relationship with food that will last for the rest of your life. By the way, this is The Way In approach to exercise as well.

It goes against our commonly-accepted knowledge—and against our never-ending quest to think up reasons we're not good enough—but the person who works out hardest or longest isn't necessarily the same one who is the leanest. In fact, that all-star workout warrior is often the person who may NEVER be svelte. Poorly strategized, overly-taxing workouts often cause people to eat amounts of food that undermine the whole reason they're working out so hard — to lose flab!

So please, close that calorie-counting app, put your fitness calculator down and make a leap of faith toward a more personalized, intuitive way of eating and exercising based on how you feel and what's true for *you*. You'll still get to log what you eat and how you move each day – how else will you know what worked and what adjustments to make as you go along? But you'll be analyzing your weekly results against yourself—your own food choices, activity levels and general life patterns—not calorie counts based on human averages or arbitrary foods chosen for you.

Metabolism is a Matter of Opinion (Your Own)

Have you ever been out with friends at a nice restaurant and eaten a so-called healthy meal—perhaps a bland salad with baked chicken and some fat-free dressing—and then as soon as you finish, you think, *Ugh, is that it? Can I order dessert now? How long until I can eat again?*

Now, calorically, that entire meal was plenty of food. There's no reason you're still hungry, except this: You *knew* it was "healthy." You didn't want the baked chicken, you wanted Frank's burger or Jill's mound of Alfredo pasta. In other words, you knew you were sacrificing something, and your hormones knew it as well.

Brain chemistry is tremendously influenced by how we view our food. Research has shown that we are more satisfied when we *believe* our meal will be satisfying.

There are two hormones at work here.

Ghrelin is the hormone in your stomach that tells your brain, "feed me!" When ghrelin levels rise, our brain lets us know it's time to find food and slows our metabolism in case we don't eat. Once we start eating, our ghrelin levels drop, which initiates the production of…

Leptin, the "I've had enough!" hormone. This hormone is not in your stomach, but in your brain, and when leptin levels rise, we know to stop eating, and our metabolism kicks into high gear.

Believe it or not, your body's hormonal "stop-eating" signals—the ones in your brain—are activated quicker when you eat food you *really like*.

What we think about our food clearly matters. Now, before you break out the triple chocolate cake, I'm not saying you'll get skinny by indulging every meal.

THE WAY IN TO YOUR BRAIN:
The Milkshake Study

NEWSFLASH: our thoughts about the yumminess of the food we eat directly influence our digestive functions, according to a study reported by Alia J. Crum, Kelly D. Brownell, and Peter Salovey of Yale University and William R. Corbin of Arizona State University (American Psychological Association, Health Psychology, May 16, 2011).

Dr. Crum's study measured participants' ghrelin levels (the *feed me!* hormone) after drinking a milkshake on two different occasions. On the first visit, people drank a shake labeled *Indulgence*, a 620-calorie decadence. One week later, they drank a shake labeled *Sensi-Shake*, a "guilt-free" 140-calorie meal replacement. What the participants didn't realize is that, on both occasions, they had been given the same exact shake. And guess what? Their hormones didn't realize it either!

Incredibly, the participant's ghrelin levels dropped almost three times more when they drank the milkshake they thought was a super-decadent, indulgent one. In other words, their body told them it was satisfied much faster when they thought they were following **The Rule of Awesome.**

If you think your meal is delicious, your hormones will help you keep your portions in control. If you are begrudgingly eating the "healthy" alternative, it most likely won't.

But I am saying that if you try to lose weight eating "diet" foods that you don't actually enjoy, it will be harder, take longer and the weight will probably creep right back on once you go back to real food. Which you will.

You Get What You Give

In my experience with clients, whatever results you achieve on quick-fix programs end up lasting for about the same length of time. Say you do some sort of 26-day "Sugar Shred." Most people will generally keep off those lost 10 pounds of flab (and muscle) for about a month. Do a five day "Carb Crusher" and keep off the few pounds of mostly water-weight you lost for about five days. Get the idea?

Of course you do, because you've done it. Over and over again. We all have. Short term "diets" end, and as soon as we get back to eating regular food on a regular schedule, we're in trouble. If you somehow haven't personally experienced this demoralizing phenomenon, you've undoubtedly seen it happen to a friend or two. Or five. Or fifty.

The fact is that pounds lost through highly restrictive plans are often not the result of lost fat, but instead the loss of water and muscle. And while we're on the topic, how gross is the idea of your body having to turn to its own muscle for fuel? These non-solutions are rarely nutritionally adequate, never realistic for a balanced life, and usually leave you with an even slower metabolism. "Crash diets" and super restrictive plans can also have a negative effect on your hormones, which don't appreciate having you playing games with them. Plus, when you do see pounds creep back up, those pounds will most likely come in the form of a new layer of fat on top of the old layer of fat you never actually lost. Short term so-called "solutions" are sooooo not worth it!

Life Happens

We are a food-loving culture. For many of us, bonding over meals is one of life's great joys. Unfortunately for people trying to lose weight, many of the meals we have with friends and family aren't in our control and aren't great for our waistline. Even when we're in a restaurant and do our best to order thoughtfully, the food is inevitably richer and saltier than we need.

Most eating programs don't take this into account. Good luck making the "plan" choice when you're staring at an endless basket of delicious, salty, house made tortilla chips. Many of the foods we enjoy with others we love for their taste, texture or sentimental reasons, and while anyone can pass on the bread basket at a restaurant once or twice, I can only think of two people in my entire career that could embrace a "No, thank you" lifestyle for the long haul. Pounds lost on a program that doesn't take into account food "peer pressure" are usually regained—and fast. People will never stop offering rich foods to us. And most of us will never stop accepting.

Likewise, we must also account for the less than advantageous food choices we make when we're celebrating, tired or stressed. Diets fail because we only temporarily realign our eating patterns while on them. The minute the plan ends, life's unpredictability often rushes us right back to sweets, bread, fried deliciousness or whatever your personal kryptonite may be.

The words *should* and *can't* don't inspire much in the way of happiness and, without joy, the changes you make won't last. If you white-knuckle your way through a diet or exercise plan, eventually you'll have to release your grip.

The Way In says yes to both social events and comfort food. There is a place for these in our lives. We allow in the extraordinary, after all! What it does not allow is mindless eating. There's a significant difference, and I'm going to help you figure out what that is. This plan is designed to not only help you comfortably hang on but to also be able to, finally, once and for all, pull yourself all the way up!

A Final Note

The fact is, by the time you find your "Way In," you won't be the same person. You're going to uncover and let out your true self—that brave, capable, visionary we all hide inside for fear of being too bold or laughed at or (gasp) failing.

So, get ready. This journey isn't easy, but I promise you, it's worth it. And most importantly, you're not alone; we're in this together. And by the way—thank you for choosing me as your guide. It's my honor.

Now get ready to impress yourself. You can do this!

THE WAY IN TO SUCCESS:
No Room for Crab Mentality

Throw a crab into a bucket, and there's a good chance she can escape. Crabs are wily, and they know how to use those pinchers. But throw that same crab into a bucket full of other crabs, and she's stuck for good. Why? In a group, the other crabs will pull down any individual that rises above the pack.

Weight loss programs are often a lot like a club—there's a group of people "in the know," and they can't wait to share their insider knowledge—with each other, with you, with the grocery clerk who mentions having arthritis. It's comforting to have parameters and rules to follow. And it can make us feel good to be on the inside.

The Way In, however, isn't a club, it's a private process. As we learn to practice personal authenticity, we need space to look inside, face our demons, and discover our strengths and weaknesses. But constant talk about how we're faring on that journey doesn't help us overcome our demons; it helps them root further into our consciousness, by feeding them with our thoughts, energy, and time. And just as importantly, it invites people in our lives to offer their own opinions. There will always be someone who thinks you can do it a better way, that self-improvement is a judgment on them, or that you'll never reach your goals. And you need those opinions about as much as you need a second helping of sheep brain casserole.

The Way In asks you to preserve your search for personal authenticity by keeping your process to yourself as much as possible. Instead of feeding your demons with talk, talk, talk, or setting yourself up for that bucket of crabs to pull you down, focus on your own journey and keep the details—as much as you can—to yourself.

4

KNOW THYSELF

WHAT KIND OF EATER ARE YOU?

OVER MY 25 YEARS IN FITNESS, I've come to know that most of us eat in a way that is completely out of sync with how our bodies work most effectively. (Myself formerly included, so definitely no judgment!)

To make this plan work effectively for life, it's important to understand how *you* operate—not your best friend, not a Kardashian, not the guy at the gym who grunts more than he sweats, not the skinny girl at yoga who apparently lives on kale pops and air. *You.*

SEE WHICH OF THESE FOOD PERSONALITY PROFILES
YOU RECOGNIZE IN YOURSELF:

When you say dinner, I say give me meat and something like a potato, grains or pasta. Maybe I'll have something green, maybe I won't. Shortly after a meal, I'm kind of tired. Sometimes (or a lot of times) I have indigestion.

The Traditionalist. You prefer big meals fewer times a day and feel pretty good about the fact that you don't really snack. Dinner is like a mini-Thanksgiving every day – you almost always have seconds. Even your smaller meals tend to be much larger than is necessary to fuel yourself until you eat again. Maybe you burp after every meal. A bunch. You feel bloated and sluggish after eating. You often need a break afterward, especially after dinner. You are intimately familiar with that "I just need to sit on the couch for a bit, so I can get to work addressing this gastrointestinal disaster" feeling.

I hardly eat, yet I'm not super slim – which is so frustrating! Seriously. I don't know what's wrong with me. And I've had my thyroid checked and my doctor says I'm fine. (I'm thinking I'll try a different doctor. Maybe someone more holistic.) I eat all good food for the most part. Except for when someone has cookies at the office or I'm at a birthday party or there are chips around. OK, I love to munch. But I'm calorie conscious and it's not like I'm eating super bad food or ginormous meals. I don't get it.

The Pick Picky. Despite rarely eating large meals, you still carry around extra weight. In your case, the problem is often that, despite your tiny meals, you consume way too many calories over the course of the day because you never feel satisfied. You keep going back for a few more bites of this. And then just a little of that. And a *tiny* taste of the other thing. And then a little more and more and even more. Picky's rarely finish processing one load of food before piling on more. Hormones that regulate hunger and digestive cues become imbalanced and can't signal properly. Once that happens, your ability to gauge food in terms of your actual energy needs doesn't stand a chance.

Sometimes I forget to eat. And honestly, I don't mind. In fact, I feel a sense of accomplishment when I forget (not that I'd ever admit it.) No, I'm not in the kind of shape I wish I was in. But skipping is at least one way I can keep enough control to stay where I'm at on the scale.

The Skipper. You feel best (you think!) when you eat very little all day, and then indulge at night. But this is totally OK by your calculations, because even when you totally binge, you're still not taking in more than 1200 calories. (That's the magic number you read somewhere, right?) You get that it would be better to take in more calories during the day when you are actually using them. But you feel that when you eat in the morning or lunchtime, it just opens the floodgates and you eat constantly for the whole rest of the day.

I eat pretty well, but I definitely munch more if I'm stressed or bummed out. Or celebrating. It's not like I use food as a reward, but I definitely like to get myself a treat at "job well done" situations. Or when someone else has a "job well done" situation. Or even just a "job done" situation. OK, I use food as both a band-aid and a reward. But whatever – it's one of life's great pleasures.

The Nervous Nelly. You basically eat pretty well… only to seriously overdo it with chips or chocolate or cocktails every time life throws us a stress-inducing curveball. And for you, curveballs seem to be life's favorite pitch. Nelly's often rationalize less than optimal food choices by telling themselves that, because of X, Y or Z, they "need it," or "deserve it," or "earned it." For you, food is both the go-to salve for life's wounds and your favorite reward when life tosses you a pitch you actually hit out of the park. Unfortunately, this is not the kind of food relationship that'll get you to the fitness championships.

I'm strong and healthy. I know what to do and I do it. When I think about it, I realize I spend a lot of my free time working out, getting or making uber-nutritious food or tooling around the internet looking for ideas about working out and getting or making uber-nutritious food. So why do I still have this layer of flab that just won't go? It's not, like, a ton, but it's more than I deserve given the time I put in and how much I know.

The Good Students. You do a whole lot right in terms of food and exercise, but you still can't seem to get that last layer of flab to pack up and leave town. Fitness-wise, you're strong and healthy. But you always seem to be doing battle with a relentless plateau. It's like your hard-earned muscles are covered in a layer of "dough" that just won't go. You like to know how you measure up against others – and you're a bit metric-obsessed in terms of food and exercise. We constantly analyze the scale and our calorie intake versus energy expenditure to the point of ignoring how we *feel* in favor of what we want numbers to show. So, you scan magazines, talk to friends, scour the internet and pay professionals for more and more and more strategies, valuations and calculations to add to your already pretty complex regimen.

I do my best thinking while chewing. I like to have food by me when I work. The End.

The Thinkers. You don't graze because you're bored or sad. You do it because you're overwhelmed with a busy mind that needs focusing. While working or even just sitting for a moment to process life, you like to pick on something "snacky" … and then on something else… and then something else. The act of chewing occupies you, quieting the loud, busy side of your brain that won't let you concentrate. You also sometimes use food to help you procrastinate. But all of this "food for thought" can cause you to suffer the same metabolic mayhem as your cousin the Pick Picky's: a physically and hormonally confused stomach that's never really fully hungry or fully empty. Also, the mindless eating you do to (ironically) quiet your mind means taking in a whole lot of unusable, extra calories.

I know I shouldn't, but I drink soda all the time. I eat candy. And chips. The fact is, I love processed food. And fast food. It's quick (duh) and easy. It keeps me going. And I honestly don't eat that much. Plus, I eat good meals at home. Don't judge me.

The Whatever. You stay at a plateau because you regularly eat processed foods like cookies, candies, chips, soda, and sugary drinks, even though the amounts you have are pretty small by your estimation. After all, what's a little bit here and there if you're eating well at night, right? (OK, wrong. And you know it.) But for whatever reason, you don't care that processed foods and drinks are made of cheap ingredients and chemicals that can seriously upset the balance of your digestive and hormonal systems if eaten regularly—even in small amounts. Or maybe you do care, but you don't have the time to change and figure out what else is as quick and easy. Whatever the reason, pass the Doritos and you'll think about it tomorrow.

SELF-KNOWLEDGE IS POWER

All seven types of misguided eating strategies lead people away from a healthy body and a lean physique, and instead result in chronic states of bloat, indigestion, inflammation, gastrointestinal distress, constipation, IBS and worst of all, *a super slow metabolism.*

How do I know this? Because I know. Personally. *Throughout my career, I have been every one of these types of eaters at different times in my life.* Sometimes in the same week! While myriad studies support my conclusions about how and why these eating behaviors negatively affect us, the most valuable lessons I have learned in my years as a fitness professional have been through my own struggles to achieve my goals.

Take it from me, an experienced fitness pro who theoretically "knew better" and still made all sorts of exercise and nutrition missteps: *achieving supreme health and a toned, lean body is not only possible, it's way simpler than you think.* But I promise you, the answer is not to be found in the latest super cleanse, diet fad or workout craze.

YOUR INNER VOICE IS RIGHT

Deep down you know the approach you've been taking isn't great and it's certainly not getting long-term, compounding results. You've experienced for years how your body has responded to the various eating patterns you've tried on only to revert back to your usual ways – what your body does in the face of inconsistency: it invites more unwanted guests to the "fat hotels" all over your body – the most prime real estate being on your belly, your hips, thighs, and back of your arms.

YOU DO YOU

We can't help but compare ourselves to everyone and everything - the celebrity in the magazine, the person on the treadmill to our left, the new hire at the office... and often, many of us actually find ourselves doing pretty well. The trouble is that we know in our hearts the "Compare Game" is one with no winner. However, in our effort to reach a personal holy grail of supremely optimal nutrition and a Nike™ commercial level of fitness, we overdo it in terms of both. Hence the never-changing flab plateau caused by an overly aggressive training regimen followed by overeating to sustain our habitual overtraining. (Which also leaves us too tired to do much else.) Too much, even of a good thing, is still too much. And we know it. But we don't know what else to do.

ALSO ALWAYS RIGHT: MOTHER NATURE

The body is designed by nature to want to live until tomorrow and has systems in place to deal with us when our mind turns us into ding-a-lings about food. Routinely skipped meals, chronic overeating and inconsistent eating are all answered with the same "two can play at that game" solution: until we get it together, our bodies slow our metabolisms to a crawl. Remember in kindergarten how when we acted out our teacher would make us put our head down on our desk until we could behave? It's kind of the same thing.

5

THE WAY IN

THE LIFESTYLE

YOU NOW HAVE MY 5 LIFE STRATEGIES, and you understand the principles behind the plan. You're well aware that the calories in/out formula is simplistic and not a very helpful guide. You know that cutting all the good food out of your life and forcing yourself to eat things you don't actually enjoy won't work. And you know that life happens.

Diet tricks don't work—but neither did the eating habits that got you off track in the first place. So, if we're not going to cut out good food, and we're not going to revert back to free-for-all dessert marathons, what are we going to change?

In a word: everything. Rather than fixing what you put into your body, we're going to fix <u>how</u> your body craves, reacts to, and processes energy. We're going to recalibrate your stomach to be full with less food at each meal. We're going to train your tongue to crave less sugar, salt and non-beneficial fats. We're going to make the best nutritional choices the no-brainer habits you can do without using up your precious willpower. And we're going to improve the way your body functions through personalized, super-efficient workouts.

There are two parts of The Way In lifestyle. The first is changing how we think about food and nutrition, which we'll talk about for the next few chapters. The second is movement and a "consistency over intensity" approach to exercise that I'll explain later in the book, along with many examples for you to try on your own.

The Goal: "Sensational" Eating

The basics of the food and nutrition part of The Way In lifestyle are simple. Rather than drastically change the food you eat, The Way In helps you be more satisfied with less (and better) food. In other words, we're going to non-surgically "shrink" your stomach. Over time, half of your usual dinner plate will be all you can finish without feeling ill. So, move the big plates to the back of the cabinet, because soon you won't know how you ever filled them up.

To achieve this, we need to get in touch with the **physical sensation** of being satiated, but not over full. Most of us are so out of touch with our own body's needs, we don't even know we've eaten until we need to unbutton the top of our pants to get comfortable. By that time, you've eaten *way* more than you need. One of the single most important lessons you will learn in this process is to put down your fork, *regardless of what is left on your plate.*

Because of this shift alone, even if you don't change the type of food you eat *at all*, you will start to lose weight. You won't be counting calories or following a strict food list, but you will be eating fewer calories, and your body will be burning them more efficiently. For the best results, however, we won't stop there—we'll retrain your body to crave less sugary, salty, processed foods and hunger for foods that are more nutritious and closer to their natural state. You won't change your eating habits out of guilt, resignation, or some sort of teacher's-pet desire to conform to rules, but because foods that are good for you are also delicious. Seriously, have you eaten a fresh peach lately? They're incredible.

The Plan

There are three parts to the nutrition side of this plan.

The first is to get your body on a schedule. Whether you're a "Traditionalist," a "Pick Pick Picky," or a "Skipper," we need to get you used to eating at regular intervals to get rid of the unpredictable highs and lows of hunger. Once you're eating the recommended number of meals a day (and that number is six—I told you this isn't about deprivation!) you will no longer swing between starving and stuffed, ensuring that you have the consistent energy you need all day long.

Next is portion modification. You may have guessed that you don't get to eat family style platter of spaghetti six times a day. But this isn't the step where you get hungry, try to power through, and eventually give up either. Over time, with the help of the simple method I've created, you will lessen the amount of food you eat at each opportunity. We'll do this slowly, so your stomach is naturally adjusting, and you still feel satisfied at meals. The key to success is that you never feel restricted or hungry when you get to dinner-time—otherwise, you'll be resentful, and your hormones will ramp up until you devour that pizza in its entirety. So, don't stress about the idea of eating less.

Eating smaller meals on a regular schedule will help you get back in tune with how your stomach actually feels—the physical sensation of hunger and satiation. You'll begin eating to fuel your body and not because it's fun or you're bored, or you need an excuse not to talk to your coworkers. That realignment is the cornerstone of becoming lean and fit for life.

The final nutrition step will be changing the food you actually eat. If there's one thing humans love almost as much as we love sugary, processed, fatty foods, it's routine. Think about what you have for breakfast every morning. It's probably the same two, maybe three dishes. Lunch is a salad or sandwich. We have a small collection of dinner options. And then our snacks—maybe it's dessert, maybe it's "Wine o'clock" every day at 7pm sharp.

We are creatures of habit, and The Way In takes advantage of this need for routine by making easy adjustments to our go-to foods. If you're going to have basically the same lunch four out of seven days a week, it might as well be one that is tasty, as close to nature as you can get, and full of the nutrients you need to thrive. The food selection portion of this plan is about putting together a roster of all-star meals that will better serve your body, called "Habit Foods." Using my simple guide, you will create a list of no-brainer Habit Foods for 80% of your meals – especially all the times you are dining alone, on the run, or just in need of something that fills you up and makes you feel good.

Remember, this is not a diet. Habit Foods aren't your new prescription, and there's no way to "fall off" or "blow it" or "be bad." What you eat doesn't define who you are. Instead, you're going to choose healthful foods for the majority of your meals.

THE WAY IN WARNING:
Beware the Good Student

Very few of my clients have a difficult time adjusting to The Way In, with one exception: the "Good Student." Always wanting to "do it the right way," this handful of people struggle with the simplicity and permissiveness of the plan. Instead, they want to go the traditional path of super-strict food rules and super-punishing workouts. Most of them have stories about that one time they were "perfect" and saw results...only to be back in my gym wondering why they couldn't stick to a plan that cut out everything good in their lives. Inevitably, those are the people who plateau quickly and stay there until they finally agree to let go of the "right way" and start listening to their bodies.

Good Students Be Warned: The Way In is going to leave a hole in your life. This plan will not torture you. It will not suck up hours of your day. And there's no gold star for suffering the most. For Good Students (myself a former member), the low overall time commitment and private, personal nature of this journey robs us of your favorite public cross to bear. But, hopefully, you'll eventually realize that the time you spent on your latest diet fad - preparing unfamiliar dishes like you're a recipe-tester for the Food Network, exercising as if you might be able to power your cell phone that way, or comparing notes on all the foods you've proudly forsaken, might just be put to better use.

In your case, dear Good Student, this is a case of **oppositional stability** – you need to take the leap to believe that less really can be more. Then, with all that extra time, attack your Life List: find a new hobby, write a book. Take a real class and be a star pupil in the literal sense. I'm not joking! Your side assignment as you follow this program is to start planning what to do with your newfound time!

Yes, you'll absolutely scarf down super-rich foods and your old favorites from time to time. I even have a name for them: "Social Foods." And guess what? Eating them is not only OK, but regular "indulgences" are precisely what make The Way In a sustainable lifestyle. Still, once your body adjusts and you're more in-tune with your stomach, you won't like how crappy you feel once you've had too much of that rich overly-sweet, or outrageously salty dish you used to love. You won't enjoy your "bad" favorites in the same way anymore. Apologies in advance (but not really).

It's All About You

These are the guidelines, and over the next few chapters, we'll get into the nitty-gritty. Each week, you'll alter one food factor and/or one movement goal at a time. By working on just one or two variables, you'll begin to understand how your body best responds to different types of food and exercise. That's the critical difference between this method and the ones you've tried before; you're learning what works for you, rather than trying to fit yourself into a plan for "average" people.

Keeping good notes during this plan will help you uncover a new Fitness Lifestyle Formula that will keep you on track forever. But remembering that "life happens" and how we all get sidelined at moments, your notes will also help deliver to you another very special bonus at the end – your personal Rapid Reset Formula.

We all need a motivational fitness "kick start" or "comeback" from time to time. One of the greatest things I do for my clients is figure out for them which combination of foods and exercise choices make them feel their leanest and strongest – their best - in the shortest amount of time. Their "Rapid Reset Formula." Confidence-building results achieved in a relatively short period can ignite that crucial spark we need to keep us fired-up on a lifetime fitness journey. Having both a Plan A and a fail-safe Plan B means never straying far from your best "you."

So, be sure to note on your LIFEtracker pages each week any days that you are feeling particularly lean, strong and full of energy. We'll discern which foods and workout choices occurred around the times you felt great and then distill them into your Rapid Reset – your personal 24-7 plan for whenever you need an extra boost toward your goals.

And remember, while I am giving you guidelines and suggestions, you are the one who will design this plan – and that's precisely why it will be sustainable for the long haul. I know you want me to tell you what to eat (all my clients beg me for that), but you'll see better results if you pick foods for yourself based on what you actually *like to eat* and find *easy to prepare* daily. Yes, it's a little more work on the front end. But if it means you'll permanently lose some of your (ahem) back end, I think we can agree that it's worth it.

My goal (and the goal of any teacher worth the price of tuition) is to help you develop unshakeable confidence, self-sufficiency and independent thinking. This plan will help you get to know yourself on a deeper level and create a way in that is entirely unique to your goals and lifestyle. After that, all you need to do is follow your own, altogether do-able plan and get ready to be done with the subject of weight loss for the rest of your life!

6

SCHEDULE: PENCIL IN YOUR SUCCESS

ALMOST EVERY CLIENT WHO COMES TO ME FOR HELP has one thing in common: They don't really know what hunger is. I was in this category myself for years. Some of them graze all day and never really get the chance to be hungry. Some of them eat so much at their three-square meals, their food isn't fully digested before they get to the next meal. Some of them skip meals all day—by accident or on purpose in a misguided desire to "be good" and shun food—only to binge as soon as the sun sets.

It isn't that they don't crave food—they crave food all the time. But usually, it's a hormonal thing, not an actual "my stomach is empty and it's time to put some food in it" thing. With the exception of my "skippers," my clients rarely ever *feel* hunger, they just *want* food. The skippers have a different kind of stomach-blindness: they feel bad, and grumpy, and sluggish, but when it comes to hunger, they only seem to know how to go from "fine" to "famished."

All of these habits end in the same result: a body that doesn't trust you and holds on to fat—either because it can't burn it, or it's convinced you might never eat again.

That's why there is no better, faster way to get the weight off your body **permanently** than to get yourself on a well-thought-out eating schedule.

Why? Because when your body expects wholesome food on a regular schedule, your body begins to trust you again, and it responds by revving up your metabolism. Your hormones will start signaling the way they should be: "feed me" when you actually need food, and "stop eating!" when you have the energy you need. Rather than never giving your body a chance to actually use the fuel you've provided it or swinging between the extremes of lethargic overeating and catastrophic starvation, your metabolism will burn consistently, with moderate fluctuations. Plus, once your schedule is set, your daily stress over when and what to eat will reduce. The math of this concept is easy: higher metabolism, consistent energy, and less stress equal a body that's primed to get lean.

Clock-watching

Rather than calorie-counting, you need to be clock-watching. Here is what you'll be watching for: Every four hours, you must eat. Sometimes you'll eat before that, but never after. This will keep your metabolism firing on all cylinders and prevent you from starvation-fueled mealtime binges. This is imperative.

For some, eating this much will be a significant adjustment, but as you follow the plan, your body will naturally be hungry every four hours. And if it isn't, you're either overeating or waiting so long that you've moved past the physical sensation of hunger. Either way, it's not good.

Four hours is your new go-without-eating limit. Even if you don't feel hungry, *and even if your next meal is coming up soon*, you must eat at least a few bites of something at the four-hour mark: a piece of fruit, a spoonful of nut butter, a bite of your leftover lunch, or a small whole-milk latte (bonus points for a plant milk with protein like hemp or oat), an ounce of dark chocolate or a cup of homemade soup. Again, it's all about a consistent schedule your body can count on.

Here is what your new schedule will look like:

A WAY IN TO SUCCESS #1:
Practice Makes Perfect Habits

As you know by now, The Way In doesn't shy away from life's food roller coaster— that's one of the reasons the Six Week Shape Up in this book is over a month long. I can promise you that, in that time, you will get broken up with via tweet, celebrate a new job, go to a wedding, a funeral or both, take a cruise, or survive the kids' schedule of 26 soccer games, 7 school projects, 12 birthday parties and one case of pink eye... or some other serious case of real-life.

The Way In doesn't just tolerate these bumps in the road it welcomes them, because there's no other way to test whether or not the habits you're building have become just that - HABITS. Remember, The Way In is not about willpower. It's about:

1. discovering what strategies are right for your body in the Six Week Shape Up, and

2. continuing to practice those strategies until they are your "new normal."

By taking the time to ingrain beneficial choices as habits, you won't be derailed by whatever adventures come your way. After that, you'll maintain your life with four, doable daily goals that make up The Way In lifestyle.

The worst thing you can do is skip ahead, get overly zealous about changing your life, and then watch all your hard work fall apart the first time you come up to those real-life hurdles. So, dive into the learning process and then trust the plan we make for you!

Breakfast

Breakfast may never be skipped. *Ever.* Each morning, your metabolism counts on you to throw a log on its fire and get it going. It is believed by some that if you don't, you will burn less and store more of every single calorie you consume for the rest of the day. There is conflicting science on whether or not skipping breakfast is detrimental to metabolism. But that's not the argument I'm making for a few bites in the morning anyway.

I believe in getting your body to be more "calorie-responsive." Developing the habit of eating food throughout the day when you need the calories and getting to know the feelings of hunger and satiety, will prevent pick-pick-picking at things throughout the day and overeating at night. Pure and simple. There are no greater tools in weight loss than eating energy-appropriate portions on a schedule in line with your energy needs. Make sense?

And never fear, as a food-on-the-run eater since forever, I'm in no way suggesting you need to get up, put on an apron and whip up a three-egg garden omelet with a side of freshly sliced strawberries every morning. (Although, the "Omelet in A Mug" recipe on my AND/life™ app will tell you how to make this a one-minute miracle). Point being, even if it's just gulping down something on the go, you must eat at least three bites of some sort of Habit Food <u>within one hour of waking up</u>.

I get it, some of you find the idea of eating something first thing in the morning a repulsive impossibility. I might as well be asking you to chew on a jellyfish and wash it down with ketchup. I'm not trying to torture you, but this is the meal that sets up your entire day. Do you really want to face that break-room coffee cake with a stomach that's roaring at you?

It doesn't have to be the second you wake up; you can wait the whole first hour to eat. If you really hate eating in the morning, just have your three bites right at the 59-minute mark. After a few days of working the plan, most people find that they can not only stomach breakfast, they wonder how they ever went without it.

If you're not opposed to the morning meal, you still might be afraid that eating first thing will "make you hungrier" throughout the day. That's the whole point. Hunger is our friend and remembering what it feels like to actually be hungry is the first step to figuring out what the appropriate amount of food is for your size and energy needs.

Mid-Morning Snack

Have a mid-morning snack within two to three hours of breakfast, but no more than four hours later. The size of it should vary based on your hunger level each day. If you ate a more substantial breakfast, have a small portion now. Or if you're particularly hungry, serve yourself a full breakfast portion (guidelines to follow). Either way, eat a little slower and stop eating the second you feel satisfied, no matter how much food is left on your plate.

The mid-morning eating time is a perfect self-teaching tool—an opportunity to listen for what your stomach is telling you about how much food it really needs at the moment. You may find the mid-morning is a hungrier time for you than you thought. Or maybe it's no biggie, requiring just three bites, so you don't end up famished at lunch. Whatever your body tells you, it's right. Do that. Just keep in mind that it may tell you something different from day to day.

Note: depending on your schedule, this meal may eventually become optional or altogether eliminated. Regardless, it's essential to start with it, in order to 1) align your food intake with your energy needs, 2) recalibrate your stomach to need less food at each meal and 3) create consistency, so your metabolism stays revved up. So, even if you don't feel hungry, have a small snack at this time for at least the first 6 weeks.

Lunch

Lunch should usually happen somewhere two and three hours after your second meal.

For some of you, there may only be four to five hours total between breakfast, mid-morning snack and lunch. Do not skip any of them. Just do your best to keep the three eating times at least two hours apart and eat only the amount of food you need to *feel satisfied* at each.

For you late-lunchers, remember the 4-hour rule. I know, I know, you're very busy, and you "forget" to eat. But we all know that you won't forget to pig out on office chips when you're crashing at 4 o'clock or eat the entire giant carton of sweet and sour chicken tonight at 9. Humans need food to function, and even the busiest, most important among us are not exempt. So, grab a sandwich (open-faced = bonus points), get a salad, have your colleague pick something up—but whatever you do, don't skip lunch!

Getting your breakfast/mid-morning/lunch routine set is the key to quick stomach recalibration. Also, by aligning your food intake with when your body actually requires more energy, you will allow your metabolic hormones to come into balance.

Afternoon snack

Here's the game-changer! In the late afternoon, get up, stretch your legs, and grab yourself a bite to eat. Even if you'll be eating dinner in an hour. This eating time is <u>crucial</u> because it boosts our energy, stabilizes our blood sugar levels and, most importantly, ensures that we don't gorge ourselves at dinner... which then opens the floodgates for all-night binge-eating to go along with whatever you're currently binge-watching.

Like breakfast, NEVER skip this one. Believe it or not, breakfast and an afternoon snack are the true keys to losing weight for good. You don't need a lot a lot of food, but you need fuel to start your day and also to power you through to the finish line. Think of it like revving your engines at the start of a race and then that crucial last pit stop before bringing it home.

The chance of overeating is highest when we are tired (i.e., after a long day of work) and/or emotional (i.e., after any given day of being alive) – and I mean this in thumbs up ways as well as thumbs down. Your exhausting day of work may have been a super-productive, inspiring, happy one. And your emotional roller-coasters du-jour may be because of a fabulous new opportunity or success—I hope they are! What I'm saying is that we can be derailed by celebrations just as easily as boo-hoo's. That's why it's so important to set yourself up to win the fitness game—no matter what your day brings—by always arriving at dinner comfortably hungry, never starving.

Dinner

If you manage to eat dinner at basically the same time every day, you're lucky. Keep it up! For everyone whose schedules change from day to day, don't worry about it. Eat your dinner when it works for you, even if it's not very long after you had your afternoon pick-me-up. And what am I going to remind you? That's right—don't wait longer than four hours. You know me so well. If you have to eat late, make sure to have something before your four-hour window closes.

Evening Snack

Almost everyone I know likes to have a little extra something at night after dinner—and guess what? That's OK! Don't deny yourself. But do me a favor and get in a little personal authenticity work first. Think about your goal to lose weight and acknowledge that you're not actually hungry (if you've followed the portion schedule, you won't be). Food after dinner is about relaxation and emotional satisfaction. By being clear with yourself about what you're doing—essentially giving yourself a food-hug at the end of the day—you will nix the need to sneak another bite... and another... and then another. Permission within guidelines is the key to avoid feeling deprived.

This goes against a lot of the so-called fitness wisdom we all seem to know. But I promise, you can have a little snack extra every single night if that's what you want and still shrink. The trick is to recognize when you go to grab that treat and find you don't actually want it. Or maybe you just want one bite. This *will* happen, on its own. Don't force it—allow for it.

Like with the mid-morning snack, learning to eat at night responsively (always asking yourself, "Do I really NEED this right now?") is an essential step on The Way In. Some days we honestly do need a little extra. Other days we don't, but we nosh anyway because it's part of our routine. Giving yourself the space to be honest about your motives and the permission to indulge within limits is the difference between a temporary, willpower-driven change and a long-term, sustainable lifestyle. That split-second check-in before each bite can make a huge difference in your life.

Feel Your Meals

In some ways, this schedule is arbitrary— "six meals a day" was not handed down to me on magical tablets by the God of Bangin' Bodies. The ultimate goal is for you to start eating within an hour of waking up and keep eating, at least every four hours when you're actually hungry. Six just happens to be the number of meals that have helped me, and my many clients get to that place.

In the next chapter, we'll discuss portion sizes and how much you should be eating at each time slot, but the most critical piece of the schedule and the following portion guidelines is to "feel your meals." Take bites when you're hungry and stop when you're not. Now, "eat when you're hungry" may not seem like revolutionary advice, but this is often one of the hardest things for people to practice.

Right from the very first week, start developing the habit of checking in with yourself as you eat. If you feel *satisfied*, <u>even if you've only taken a few bites</u>, stop eating that second. Take your food for later or throw it away rather than overeat. I don't want you to be wasteful for the rest of your life, but "starving kids in whichever country" weren't going to finish your salad anyway. We're burning your Clean Plate Club membership card today.

After you finish, check the time and immerse yourself in work or fun or whatever for two hours. Once the time has passed, start checking in with your stomach for *honest sensations* of hunger. Ideally, as your metabolism starts to hum along, this will happen somewhere between 2-4 hours later.

Don't just eat because two hours is up. The two-hour mark is the point where your previous, properly portioned meal will be almost, if not wholly, digested. Your hormones will come into play and help you know when it's time for the next meal. Pay attention to your body, wait for cues and then honor them.

Remember when you were a kid, and you would play and play until you felt hungry? You'd eat something, and then go back to playing...until you felt hungry again. That kind of intuitive, responsive relationship between you, your stomach and the exciting things you want to do with your time is what we're going for. You're getting back in touch with your body. And now that you're on a schedule, it will free up your time. Instead of sitting and eating, or sitting and *thinking* about eating, you can focus on more interesting, important parts of your life.

THE WAY IN TO YOUR BRAIN:
The Zeigarnik Effect

Humans are hard-wired to seek completion. If there's one thing that gets under our collective skin, it's loose ends. We all struggle with things that are left half-done. They sit there, in the front of our minds, sucking up mental energy and bugging us until we finally give them our attention.

In the 1920's, Russian psychologist Bluma Zeigarnik conducted a series of experiments in which she concluded that unfinished tasks are imprinted in the front of the memory and remain there until they are resolved. Like a hangnail, incomplete things constantly remind us of their presence, causing discomfort and distraction. In terms of food, when a plate is piled high, our natural inclination for closure goes from inkling to imperative.

Further, as each of us juggles more and more unfinished tasks—texts unanswered, emails unopened, plans unfinalized—it's not surprising that a plate of food becomes a sort of mental oasis, a task we can fully and quickly "accomplish." So even if you're full, the Zeigarnik Effect means you'll most likely finish whatever plate is in front of you.

We can't just blame our moms forever. Part of the cleaning our plate thing is 100% on us. Get in the habit of keeping your plates manageable and practice this essential mental skill: Being OK with the "unfinished business" of an uneaten food.

7

RECALIBRATE TO LIBERATE

YOU NOW KNOW WHEN TO EAT—the next question is how much? Believe it or not, the secret to lean is in the palm of your hands!

Place your hands side by side on the table, thumbs together, fingers loosely apart. This square is a basic blueprint of the ideal size of a lunchtime or dinnertime meal. (For some people, this is the size of breakfast, too.) This square—your hands—is not a tower. It's not even a house. It's just a square, single layer of food.

For example, a lunch or dinner portion would look like this:

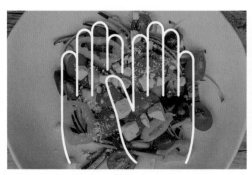 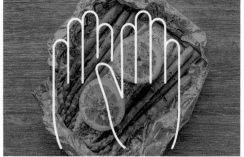

It would completely fill a salad plate or, as you can see here, the center of a dinner plate. Now, if you are hyperventilating at the idea of this being a meal, please don't freak out. I realize that, for some of you, this may seem like the amount of food you'd offer a stray kitten. There are three things you need to know right now:

1. Your stomach will slowly calibrate down to a meal this size.

2. Your hand portion is just starting place. Knowing that you will most likely finish whatever you put in front of you, the idea is to create a natural stopping place for at least a 10-minute break. Some days you may still be hungry and will eat up to another single hand-sized portion of your meal or a few bites of any Habit Food. But more often, you will be surprised to find that you actually feel satisfied and can go the recommended 2-4 hours without more. This point bears repeating: *I will never ask you to go hungry.*

3. The best part of this strategy is yet to come.

For portioning into bowls, a good rule of thumb is to think of one hand equaling one cup and testing it out. Measure water into one of your own bowls to get a sense of what one and two cup portions of food would look like. For salads, try putting one cup of your veggies in the bottom of the bowl and then filling with greens the rest of the way. A satisfying serving of pasta or chili might start out being more for you than two cups but will probably end up being about that once your stomach calibrates down. Bowls are an eyeball situation until your stomach can be relied upon to give you fullness cues – and you can be relied upon to listen to them!

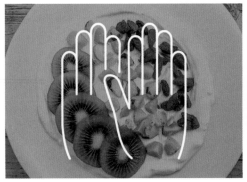 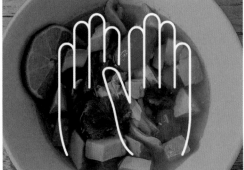

(FYI, the good part is still coming. Keep going.)

Look at one of your hands. Your hand is about the right size for you as a snack. A medium sized apple would fit into your hand. As would one or two hard-boiled eggs, a half of a nut butter and pure fruit spread sandwich (a "clean" PB&J), a piece of rolled up string cheese, five or six bites of leftover dinner or lunch, a small yogurt… You get the idea. And if you don't, you will.

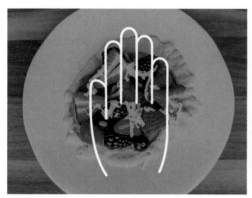 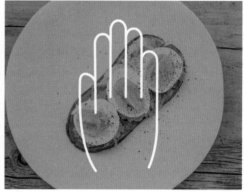

OK, seriously—stop freaking out. I know, these portions might seem *crazy small*. You might feel like you'd get more to eat as a contestant on Survivor. But like I said in the last chapter, your stomach needs to "empty out" between meals and snacks so you can get back in touch with what it is to be hungry. For real. Before every meal, your stomach should be saying, "I'm empty. Let's eat.," rather than your brain saying "I'm bored. Let's eat…" or your heart saying, "I'm lonely. Let's eat…" or your nerves saying, "I'm stressed. Let's eat."

I have never had a client for whom a one- or two-hand portion of food wasn't enough in the first few weeks of this program or training with me. It's crucial that you never leave a meal unsatisfied. If you are truly hungry after your scheduled one- or two-handed portion, go have another few bites. But before you do, please get active and DO SOMETHING for ten minutes (how about that Life List?) to see if it truly *is* hunger. As this program goes on, adding activity to your day and intensifying workouts, there will be times you do need a few bites more - and you will be able to trust that you are actually hungry and enjoy the extra food. But for right now, get ready to surprise yourself with how little food you really need each time you sit down to eat.

The Right Size at the Right Time

If you want to achieve and maintain a slimmer, healthier self forever, "eyeballing" your food against your own hands will give you a simple, new baseline portion to start with at any one sitting. And if you honestly need to eat more, you will. Moreover, every two to four hours, you'll have the chance to eat something else that's awesome, so there's never a reason to feel deprived.

Now that you know how portioning works, let's put it together with the schedule.

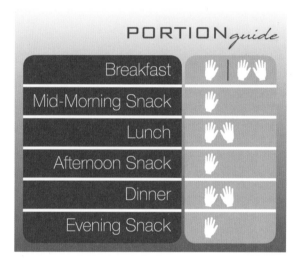

As I described earlier, some meals are flexible. For example, breakfast may be either one- or two-hands depending on your schedule and what you can stomach. Do either a one-hand breakfast and a one-hand mid-morning snack OR have a two-hand breakfast and maybe skip a morning snack if you have lunch within four hours.

Lunch and dinner are two hands. Snacks are all one hand.

Easy, right?

This schedule isn't set in stone for life — it's a tool to help you design your best lifestyle. For example, you may end up eating meals closer together on random "hungry days" or during the first weeks of this program than will feel right by the end. You might opt for a one-hand breakfast on workdays but have a two-hand breakfast on weekends. Likewise, for the evening snack –you may have days that you don't want anything. That's fine as long as you're not ignoring your body's messages.

Honor your hunger. Let it tell you when you need fuel. If it's telling you to have another portion, especially in the early days, that's totally fine. If you need to add a small one-handed snack to make it to your next two-handed meal, that's OK. This is a process. But know that the goal you are working toward is a personalized schedule of five to six meals a day, that includes no more than three two-hand size portions – that's the permanent lifestyle.

And yes, die-hard Calorie Counters out there, you're correct. All foods are not the same. But take a chill pill for just a minute, because with a recalibrated stomach and newly responsive metabolism, this is all going to equal out in the end.

Relish your personalized portions—allow in the extraordinary!—and remind yourself that you never need to eat past the point of "satisfied."

SELF-CHECK

Here's how to figure out the difference between satisfied and full:

- **When you've eaten enough, you can immediately move on to another activity.**

- **When you're full, you feel sluggish and need a break "to digest."**

If leaving a few bites on your plate sounds like a challenge to you right now, don't worry. It won't be for long. Using your own hands as a guideline, you will develop the *habit* of checking in with yourself and familiarize yourself with the feeling of satisfaction. Being full will no longer be a feeling you tolerate and will become a state you want to avoid. You'll be shocked by how content you feel with the amount of food your hands guide you to eat – and how horrible you feel when you go past that. And with easily digestible meals, your metabolism will kick into high gear, and you'll feel better all around.

As an added bonus, many of my clients find that seemingly "chronic" digestive troubles vanish on this plan, revealing that the issue wasn't a food sensitivity or allergy after all. That doesn't mean you should self-diagnose or skip seeing your doctor if you think something's up! Some digestive issues

A WAY IN TO SUCCESS #2:
Keep Your Machine Running Well

Imagine a high-tech washing machine—the newest model, with all the bells and whistles. It weighs your clothes and knows the right speed, it adds the fabric softener at just the right time, and it's super water and energy efficient. Now imagine you try to fit all of your clothes in at once. The dirtiest ones. You can barely shut the lid, you've stuffed it so full. How well is that advanced machine going to clean your clothes now?

Your stomach is similar—it's efficient, smart, perfectly attuned to your needs. Every time you eat, it breaks down food in three ways:

Mechanically - physical action of the stomach churning

Chemically - the release of enzymes and hydrochloric acid to break down food

Hormonally – the control of churning, digestive juice release, acid balance

Your stomach is capable of doing complex work, but if you stuff it full of food, it can't do its job right. Ironically, when we overeat, our machine halts to a crawl just to be able to handle all we've put in it, it takes longer to digest our food and our metabolism slows. That's why it's crucial to know the difference between your personal feelings of satisfied and full.

You know those couple extra bites of food we don't really want or need, but shove down anyway just because they're there? (Zeigarnik effect, anyone?) Visualizing your stomach overfull and unable to churn may just help you resist eating what you don't want or need. And every time you pass on that extra two or three bites, you move two or three steps closer to your goal!

are genetic or conditions that need to be managed with the help of a doctor. And sometimes foods simply don't work for us... like how I can't eat raw kale or more than five almonds without suffering in some incredibly unattractive ways. But many digestion issues are caused by our own habits—in other words, indigestion. If there's too much food in your stomach for enzymes and acids to break everything down properly, your metabolism is being sabotaged right from the beginning.

How to Get Started: At the End

Dinner is often people's favorite meal of the day, but it's also the most challenging when we're trying to honor our health goals. This is usually the time when we are tired and/or emotional from our day, we have to navigate different preferences, and it's a meal that is traditionally the biggest. For all of those reasons, I find it's the best one to begin to learn about our food habits.

So, when you serve dinner tonight, do me a favor: make yourself a plate as you normally would and then push all your food into the center. Yes, it's a strange favor. Just work with me.

OK, let's assess: Would your two hands cover the portion of food you served? If not, how much more did you serve yourself? One hand more? Two hands more? Just notice. Try not to judge. It's information.

Now, let's find you a new dinner portion starting point. Whatever food on your plate extends beyond a two-hand portion, spoon the extra into a separate small container right now and put it away in the fridge for later. Once you've finished your new portion of dinner, stop and self-evaluate. Give yourself ten minutes. If you are still hungry, go get that extra portion and eat it without guilt. But even that short pause gives your stomach a chance to readjust. We're drawing a line between mindless Zeigarnik-effect eating and food you actually need.

And here's the thing: Some nights you will genuinely be hungry for more. Maybe on day one. But soon, that ten minutes will pass, and you'll have moved on. When you are hungry again, you can go back to that meal, or you might want something different. It's all permissible. The point is that you will most likely be eating again tonight, so there's no need to worry about missing out on those last bites.

The Good Part!

Alright, you've stuck with me this far, and now it's time for the good news you've been waiting for. I've alluded to it before, but to be 100 percent clear: No food is off limits. It's true.

By getting a handle on the *quantity* of food you eat, you can stop feeling bad about *what* you're eating.

Why? In an effort to "be good," we spend so much brain power judging every bite that we eat. Our running tally of victories (egg whites and dry toast for breakfast is a "yay!") and missteps (brownies at the office party is a "boo!"), leaves us feeling like failures. Self-shaming is not helpful to weight-loss—in fact, it might be why you've got excess weight in the first place!

This is the point in the plan where my clients tell me to cut the crap and tell them what they should *really* eat. And perhaps, you're thinking, "I'm not a dummy, Andrea, I know I'm not going to lose weight eating ice-cream all the time." Yes, I know, you want to lose weight and you want it off right now, right now, *right now*!

But listen—and I'm really serious about this—you've got to relax. Stress makes your body treat fat like a life preserver on the stormy sea of your own self-loathing—there's no way in hell it's letting go. Scarcity—the perception that we are lacking something we desperately need or want—is one of the most counter-productive places from which we can operate. And the number one way to make yourself feel the dread of scarcity (besides signing up for one of those survival reality shows) is to set a limit to the food you are allowed (calorie tracking) or create a list of all the foods you can't have (elimination diets). Even restriction diets that are nutritionally sound can wreak emotional havoc by making you feel like you must continually deny your needs.

If you want to eliminate foods from your diet, the only way it will ever work for the long haul is if it stems from a deep principle (i.e., "I don't eat veal because I think it's torture") or a health crisis ("I don't eat dairy because I'm severely lactose intolerant"). "I don't eat birthday cake because I would like to wear a smaller pant size" is not going to cut it. Unless you have a deep-seeded reason, inspired by your head and heart rather than your mirror, food elimination diets will leave you vulnerable to motivation-destroying self-judgment whenever we give in to our urges.

A WAY IN TO SUCCESS #3:
Embracing Dinner Again

There's probably not a meal we associate more with our emotions than dinner. It's when we connect with our fellow diners, tell stories, share our tragedies and triumphs, laugh, argue, decompress, judge, soothe—whether that's all with our families and friends or characters on a TV show (no shame, we all eat in front of the TV at times). Dinner is how we begin the close-out process for each day.

Which is great—except when we're "dieting." Like me, you've probably had those panicked diet-dinner thoughts when you realize it's your last meal on the plan for the day... OMG - is this really all I get to eat? Am I going to get enough? Is this sad, tasteless "healthy" food substitute really my reward for a hard day of living? This is rabbit food. Which might be fine for rabbits, but maybe that's because rabbits don't have it as hard. And on and on...

The Way In alleviates this anxiety by saying dinner doesn't have to be the last meal of your day. And you don't have to conform to unrealistic food restrictions that make you feel stressed or isolated from the people you're dining with. What it does ask you to let go of is the idea that this meal has to be a feast. And if you're eaten on schedule for the rest of the day, the two-hand portion should be enough to satisfy you—the trick is giving yourself time to notice.

So instead of stressing about what and when you're going to eat, approach dinner as a time to allow in the extraordinary by doing the following:

Slow down. Chew your food. Savor every bite of your non-dietized, real, delicious food.

Put down your fork at least five times. (Yes, I just made that number up. But now it's in your head and you'll think about it.) The real point is to use dinner time to talk to your companions. Ask questions and really listen to their answers! If you're eating alone, sit back and take in whatever you are doing—decompressing about your day, watching a great show, or reading a book.

When you finish, stop. Seriously, stop. And change the atmosphere - clean the dishes, walk the dog, do a crossword puzzle on your phone. Check the clock before you start and give yourself ten full minutes before you think about your stomach again. If you can do it, determine to wait a half hour. (Most likely by then, you'll get involved in something and forget for much longer than that.)

Restricting calories is a similarly unfeasible approach to weight loss because our hunger changes from day to day. The worry forces us into over-drive to find a way to satisfy our discomfort. Here's a typical scenario: even though you are pretty hungry, you eat very little (or try not to eat at all) for as long as you can... until you eventually say, "screw it" and binge on a bag of chips. Sound familiar? You and I both know it does. Because we've done it many, many, many times... Ugh.

So, from now on, we're going to skip the side of "judgment sauce."

It really doesn't matter what I eat?

No. It does. You know it does. But, *HOW* you approach food matters even more.

Some foods are highly advantageous to us: veggies, fruits, lean proteins, legumes, whole grains, etc. Some foods are less so: cookies, potato chips, Fettuccine Alfredo. And some foods are not really food at all - and you know exactly what I mean - but we sometimes eat them anyway.

Obviously, if all of your meals are made up of the latter category, you are not going to lose weight, and you're certainly not going to be enjoying a body that functions at its best. You know all of this.

What matters more *right now,* however, is <u>when</u> you eat and <u>how much</u>. That's our first order of business in Week One of the Six Week Shape-Up in this book. By tackling the issue of meal timing and food portions first, you will establish habits that both rev up your metabolism and create fat-melting calorie control, without the anxiety of calorie counting or food elimination.

In Week Two, we'll establish a variety of guideline-chosen, nutritious "Habit Foods" that will become the cornerstones of your new lean lifestyle. These will be highly beneficial, minimally processed, low sugar, low sodium, easy to make, no-brainer, go-to foods that you will eat at least 80% of the time—not out of guilt or shame, but because you like them, and they make your life easier.

But, I am still not going to tell you not to eat *anything*. On the right day, I, your fearless guide to fitness, will still eat the heck out of an Almond Joy. And I don't think twice about it while I'm licking chocolate off my fingers.

THE WAY IN TO SUCCESS #4:
Think Twice Before Eliminating Foods

Unless you have a medically-diagnosed issue or strong personal belief, never eliminate entire food groups from your diet. If your doctor advises you not to eat any red meat, please listen to her or him. If you honestly don't feel so great anytime you eat gluten, absolutely adjust. If you feel deep down in your soul that dairy should only be eaten by baby cows, honor that conviction.

Every other Tuesday, it seems we're frightened into eliminating something entirely from our diet for reasons that may or may not apply to us. Please don't make sweeping changes to your life because it's what the skinny girl on the spinning bike next you said she does or because People magazine says that's how Ryan Reynolds got ripped for his last movie. None of that (if it's even true) has anything to do with you.

Haphazard food elimination is, at best, a well-intentioned personal science experiment and, at worst, a socially annoying act of culinary narcissism. Many chronic digestive troubles can be significantly eased, if not completely eliminated, simply by eating smaller, appropriate portions of food on a regular schedule and taking a daily probiotic. A moderate approach to food may not be the kind of sexy, catchy, magical approach you see all over the internet these days . But it really can work wonders.

Believe it or not, in terms of sheer weight loss, the *what* you eat isn't as important as the *how* you eat. Once you get the scale moving downward and your self-confidence moving upward, we'll work on optimal nutrition. So, let's focus on the *how* — meal portions and timing — and get some pounds off for good!

8

HEALTH IS NOT AN ACT —IT'S A HABIT

DURING YOUR FIRST FEW DAYS OF THE WAY IN, you will focus on just two things: getting on a schedule and changing your portions. You do not need to adjust any of the types of foods you are eating.

HABIT FOODS

So you keep talking about it - what the heck is a Habit Food already?

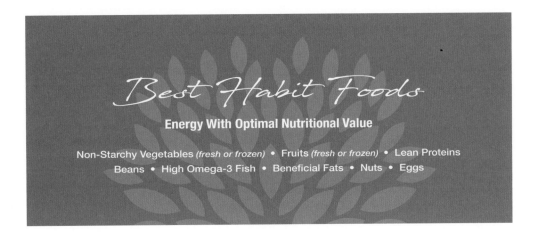

Best Habit Foods

Energy With Optimal Nutritional Value

Non-Starchy Vegetables *(fresh or frozen)* • Fruits *(fresh or frozen)* • Lean Proteins
Beans • High Omega-3 Fish • Beneficial Fats • Nuts • Eggs

Imagine a tree in the center of a beautiful field – long branches reaching, green leaves swaying in the breeze, animals playing. Life happens here. The image of this tree represents foods in their most natural state—berries, nuts, asparagus…OK, asparagus doesn't grow on trees. And neither does chicken or fish, which also happen to be up in my tree, but I think you get my drift. It's nature's best foods—simple, whole and super-nutritious:

- Non-starchy vegetables

- Fruit

- Lean proteins, including eggs

- Fish, especially high Omega-3

- Beneficial fats, like oils from nuts, seeds, olives, and coconut

- Nuts

- Beans

These foods are your <u>Best Habit Foods</u>. Eat these at every meal, and your body will thank you.

If you're confused by the addition of nuts and fats, don't be. Current science recognizes the value of high-quality saturated fats in our diets in actually protecting our heart and brains and staving off cancer. The fats and oils that come from nuts and certain plants (i.e., avocados, olives, grapeseed) are a necessary addition to your Habit Foods list. Also, although calorie-dense, high quality fats create feelings of fullness and satiety that are crucial in helping you ratchet your portion sizes down to suit your actual energy needs. See my Beneficial Fats Cheat Sheet in **Chapter 13** for guidance.

As you continue down the tree, and you enter another section: <u>Limited Habit Foods</u>. These are also healthful, wholesome foods, and they are an essential part of a healthy lifestyle. But most likely, you aren't going to be able to maintain a healthy weight and achieve optimal nutrition if you are eating cheese six times a day. It's just not going to happen.

As Habit Foods, these foods can absolutely be incorporated into your roster of go-to meals. However, these foods tend to be energy-dense, meaning they provide a lot of calories that don't necessarily make you feel full. It's really easy

Best Habit Foods

Energy With Optimal Nutritional Value

Non-Starchy Vegetables *(fresh or frozen)* • Fruits *(fresh or frozen)* • Lean Proteins
Beans • High Omega-3 Fish • Beneficial Fats • Nuts • Eggs

Limited Habit Foods

**Energy With High Nutritional Value,
But Limit To Two Servings Or Less Each Day**

Starchy Vegetables • Dairy & Cheese • Whole Grains • Honey and Pure Maple Syrup
Nut or Plant-Based Milks • All-Natural Dark Chocolate
High Quality Bars and Protein Powders • Red Meat *(2 per week)*

to get more energy than you need with Limited Habit Foods. Some of these foods are processed (whole grain foods, high quality bars, protein powders) which is what puts them a step below Best Foods. Also, this group includes otherwise beneficial foods that can nonetheless lead to inflammation or other systemic issues (dairy and red meat). For these reasons, Limited Habit Foods should only be eaten one or two times a day:

- Starchy vegetables like potatoes and beans

- Whole dairy products like cheese, plain yogurt, butter, and milk

- Whole grain foodsHoney and natural maple syrup

- High-quality fruit/nut bars

- Protein powders

- Dark Chocolate

- Red meats (only 2x or less per week)

Limited Habit Foods might be slightly processed — some of these foods have to come in packages. Unless you're my Dad and his wife Nancy, you're not going to bake your own bread and muffins every time. Unless you're my brother, you're not going to tap a tree for maple syrup. Ok, my brother's never done that. But he's incredibly handy and resourceful and if I was camping (unlikely) and forgot the syrup for breakfast pancakes (probable), he's the guy who would get some tool from his truck and make the magic happen.

Anyway, the point is that packaged Limited Habit Foods must be the best of the bunch. They are free of additives, preservatives, unpronounceable extras and never "diet-ized" to lower natural sugar or fat content.

Preparation of your Habit Foods is crucial. They should be prepared only by:

- Baking

- Broiling

- Grilling

- Poaching

- Slow Cooking

- Pressure Cooking

- Sautéing in beneficial oil

- Roasting in beneficial oil

SOCIAL FOODS

Once we leave our tree, we venture down into the world of Social Foods. This is where things get dicey.

How you handle Social Foods will either make or break your fitness journey and prospects for long-term success.

My 20+ years of experience as a fitness professional (and my 40+ years of experience as a human) has taught me that any fitness strategy that doesn't make room for Social Foods is completely unrealistic for the long-term. My strategy is to divide Social Foods by nutritional benefit – Preferred Social

Foods have some and Low Value Social Foods are basically a waste. Not a never. But, calories to be reserved only for moments of acute depression, late-night college-style eating, kid's birthday parties, run-ins with the Easter Bunny and Halloween.

Best Habit Foods

Energy With Optimal Nutritional Value

Non-Starchy Vegetables *(fresh or frozen)* • Fruits *(fresh or frozen)* • Lean Proteins
Beans • High Omega-3 Fish • Beneficial Fats • Nuts • Eggs

Limited Habit Foods

Energy With High Nutritional Value, But Limit To Two Servings Or Less Each Day

Starchy Vegetables • Dairy & Cheese • Whole Grains • Honey and Pure Maple Syrup
Nut or Plant-Based Milks • All-Natural Dark Chocolate
High Quality Bars and Protein Powders • Red Meat *(2 per week)*

Preferred Social Foods

Energy With Some Nutritional Value And Some Detrimental Factors

Organic Dairy Products with Added Sugar • High Quality Bread & Pasta
Organic/All-Natural Packaged Foods • Juice, Wine

Let's start with Preferred Social Foods, the type that are still high-quality and have nutritional value. They may be the exact same foods that are in the tree, it's just that preparation or processing bumps them out of the Habit Foods category. Think richer dishes you get at a restaurant or when friends have you to dinner. Even if you're sure the food is thoughtfully sourced and prepared with wholesome ingredients, you still can't be 100% sure what exactly is in your meal. But what you can be sure of is that you're being served more sugar and salt than you use in your quick Habit Food recipes. That's just how we cook for guests. Once you give that fact a hug, you're on your way to a lifetime fitness solution.

- Foods prepared at a quality restaurant, bakery, or friend's home
- High-quality whole grain pasta and bread
- Cane Sugar
- Dairy products with sugar added, like yogurt, gelato, and all-natural ice cream
- Wine and Juice
- Organic frozen meals

The addition of sugar, salt or natural ingredients required for processing are what separate these foods that still have nutritional value from Habit Foods.

Perhaps you're looking at this list and saying, *OK fine … but wait… juice?!* Yes. Juice. Even the all-natural stuff. Juice is all the sugar (fructose) of fruit but with none of the insulin-moderating fiber. Instead, get your vitamin C from an actual whole piece of fruit – or better yet, broccoli!

Head even further down away from the tree and you'll get to Low-Value Social Foods, our last (and, in this case hopefully "least" in terms of your diet) section.

To be honest, I'm not sure we can call all the items in this section "food." This group includes things that come in a box or wrapped in plastic and feature strange, alien ingredients and colors like "traffic cone orange." They are full of poly-syllabic ingredients that you can't pronounce without a PhD.

- Fried foods
- Bleached flours
- Packaged Foods
- Dried Fruit

- Juice

- Soda

- Hard alcohol and mixers

- Blended drinks

- Foods with trans fats

- Foods with lots of unpronounceable additives.

All of that said, here's the thing: these Low-Value Social Foods are only that – low value. This doesn't mean they are totally off-limits.

WHAT?? You're saying eat the Twinkie?

In short, yes.

Not often. Preferably never. But, this is about reality. Constant judgment about the food we eat in terms of "good" and "bad" is getting us nowhere. Instead of giving foods powerful black and white labels of good and bad (and labeling ourselves the same way when we eat them), start to think of all foods in terms of specific *benefit*. This will take the emotional charge out of eating and unlock the door to being lean forever.

One goal of creating a rotation of no-brainer Habit Foods you eat 80% of the time is to take power away from Low-Value Social foods. Knowing that you are "allowed" to eat them helps reduce their tractor-beam pull on you. Between this permission and your changing tastes, you will eat low-benefit items less often. Much less often. Many of them almost never.

So, if you just *love* potato chips or little doughy white bread rolls at restaurants or sugar-laden trail mix sold at gas stations, then follow the Rule of Awesome and eat them in small amounts as part of your Social Foods. You will gain zero benefit physically, but you'll find that Low-Value Social Foods won't cost you much fitness-wise either when eaten mindfully as part of a total life strategy. Plus, you will benefit mentally by eliminating obsessive thinking patterns around "bad" foods you ate and therefore have "blown it" or that you didn't eat and so instead gorged yourself on piles of "good foods" in an attempt to feel satisfied.

THE WAY IN WARNING:
When Bad Things Happen to Good Fruits

Before you try to be "good" by eating nothing but a big fruit salad, read this:

Fructose is the sugar that makes fruit so delicious. It's good for energy, but not everyone is good at digesting it. Your ability to process fructose is dependent on the number of GLUT5 receptors you have in your small intestine. It is through these transporters that fructose makes its way to the liver to become potential energy either in the form of glycogen or fat. When there is more fructose present than you have transporters for, all that leftover fruit sugar has no choice but to wander its way on down to your large intestine and wreak havoc.

Dumping too much fruit sugar into the gut is like spinning the wheel of fortune at the Abdominal Fun-Times Carnival. When excess fructose hits the large intestine, it's quickly fermented by hungry bacteria, resulting in gas, bloating, and abdominal pain. Fructose draws water into the intestine which, for some people, then causes diarrhea. Other side effects are cramping and constipation. Extra fructose, like all sugar, is eventually transformed into fat as well. Because fruit is different for everyone, we all need to practice personal authenticity and find out what that means for us as individuals.

During week five of the Shape-Up, you will test one-hand portions of fruit as snacks to see how/if they negatively affect your digestion.

So, wait… is fruit good for me? Yes! Fruit is very nutritious. But it's important to find out how much of a "good thing" is still a good thing for you personally.

Best Habit Foods

Energy With Optimal Nutritional Value

Non-Starchy Vegetables *(fresh or frozen)* • Fruits *(fresh or frozen)* • Lean Proteins
Beans • High Omega-3 Fish • Beneficial Fats • Nuts • Eggs

Limited Habit Foods

Energy With High Nutritional Value, But Limit To Two Servings Or Less Each Day

Starchy Vegetables • Dairy & Cheese • Whole Grains • Honey and Pure Maple Syrup
Nut or Plant-Based Milks • All-Natural Dark Chocolate
High Quality Bars and Protein Powders • Red Meat *(2 per week)*

Preferred Social Foods

Energy With Some Nutritional Value And Some Detrimental Factors

Organic Dairy Products with Added Sugar • High Quality Bread & Pasta
Organic/All-Natural Packaged Foods • Juice, Wine

Low-Value Social Foods

Energy With Low Nutritional Value And A High Level Of Detrimental Factors

Sausage & Cured Meats • Packaged Foods with Chemical Preservatives • Non-Beneficial Fats
Fried Foods • Bleached Foods *(i.e., foods made with white flour)* • Canned Foods High In Sodium
High Fructose Foods Including Syrups, Nectars & Dried Fruits • Hard Alcohol

The fact is, portions are the name of the game. When you ratchet down your stomach size on this plan, you can get away with a lot more than you think - especially with your personal Habit Foods strategy in place to guarantee highest-level nutrition every single day. And within a week or two of the plan, you WILL begin to choose Low-Value Social Foods less and less often and in smaller and smaller amounts. You just will. Super-salty, sugary, fatty, chemical-laden foods simply won't be as pleasurable anymore.

Low-Value Social Foods also include basically all caloric drinks except for juice, wine, milk and preferred plant-based milks. Getting to your fitness goals isn't just about food, it's also about what you drink. For example, a large blended coffee, tea or cocktail or two can easily give you half, if not almost an entire day's worth of calories in just one sitting. This is simply too much energy to lose weight and keep it off – and remember, this energy comes without nutritional value or feelings of fullness. I'll dive deeper into hydration and a guideline for drinks in a moment, but for the most part, most caloric drinks should be considered Social Foods. There are three exceptions which all count as Limited Habit Foods:

- Milk or plant-based milk in coffee (a reasonable splash, not a latte's worth)

- Oat, hemp or other plant milk with big protein, fiber and vitamins: one cup = one-hand

- Red wine, which has proven health benefits: 86 oz = one serving (But make the switch to 6oz servings at home and you'll save yourself 10 pounds worth of calories in a year!)

If you're wondering where artificial sweeteners like saccharin (Sweet'N Low), aspartame (Equal) and sucralose (Splenda) go on this list, it's nowhere. I promised you that no food was off limits, but these chemicals are not food and should not be a part of your diet, ever. There is a mountain of information surrounding potentially damaging effect of artificial sweeteners, most upsettingly, that they affect your brain's response to food and are linked to obesity. You might as well just eat the sugar.

THE WAY IN TO SUCCESS #5:
Public Enemies 1 & 2

SUGAR gives us quick energy (as opposed to the slower burn of fat) but it also makes our bodies dump insulin. This begins a terrible cycle where our bodies:

1. Stop burning fat because we have SO. MUCH. ENERGY!!!!
2. Quickly burn through said energy.
3. Immediately crave the fast, easy energy of more sugar.

And any energy left over immediately becomes fat. That's true of all sugars, even natural ones, even plain fruit. But much worse are concentrated forms of fructose (i.e., high-fructose corn syrup), which is more likely than sucrose (cane sugar) to harm your health by clogging your arteries with plaque.

SALT helps regulate your body's fluid levels. Too much of it causes your blood vessels to hang on to extra water, putting pressure on the walls of those vessels like turning up the water flow on a hose. When you push around all that extra blood, you essentially work your heart to death. Yeesh. That's why high blood pressure, the number one risk factor for US women's deaths and number two for men, is called the "silent killer."

But never fear: your personally authentic Habit Food strategy limits the amount of sugar and salt you eat without you even thinking about it AND changes your tastes away from them without you realizing it. You'll want less not because I recommend it (I do), or because the American Heart Association recommends it (they do), but because your taste buds will say, "no thanks."

9

HABIT FOODS HOW-TO'S

Putting Together Your Habit Foods List

IN THE FIRST THREE DAYS OF THE PROGRAM, you'll address only food portions and eating schedule. You won't change a single food you eat and don't be surprised if you lose a quick pound or two just from this.

In Chapter 11 you will find Habit Food worksheets with sections for each of your daily meals. In those sections, you will find lines for regular Habit food options and also a couple of Best Habit Food only options for times when you need to eat super clean. Each week throughout the Shape-Up, you will be told what kind of food ideas to find and add to these lists. Make the process easier at the start by simply tweaking some meals you already eat regularly to fit Habit Food guidelines. Coming up with all new things every week for every single meal is a lot.

Never fear, if coming up with food ideas sounds harder than doing the crossword in the Sunday New York Times, there are gazillions of ideas on my AND/life app. Whatever you come up with, they should be recipes that are easy to make or throw together on the fly and that you look forward to eating. The idea is to make your foods more beneficial and your life easier at the same time, not to put you through cooking school. And, please do not start forcing down kale salads every day at lunch because you think that's what skinny people eat.

Everyone always wants to know what I eat, so here's a peek into my current rotation. But please keep in mind, this is what works for me. And only right now. I will get bored of these foods and, one at a time, switch them out for different things. Four months ago, a lot of these foods were different choices.

Also, these may not be foods that excite you. It's crucial to do your own thing within Habit Food guidelines and come up with meals and snacks that suit your tastes. Please don't blindly follow what I do and turn my whole program into just another "diet" – it would defeat the purpose of you figuring yourself out, and we'd just be walking the same worn path you've already tried so many times that gets you nowhere. So OK... with all those disclaimers here goes:

Like many of you, my life is extremely busy, and my schedule is always changing. I need to have foods I can toss together fast, take with me to eat on the run, or find at restaurants easily. Here are the foods in my current breakfast & lunch rotation:

BREAKFAST

- Two mini egg frittatas1/2 Nut-butter sandwich using pure-fruit spread on whole-grain bread

- Bircher Meusli

LUNCH

- Open-faced turkey sandwich with random veggies and smashed avocado for "mayo"

- Roasted chicken and avocado with hot sauce or over greens with lemon and olive oil

- One over-easy egg with broccoli or asparagus sautéed in olive oil

Those are my go-to's. I don't spend a half hour with the refrigerator door open, debating between any number of food choices, picking at a little of this and a little of that while I think about it (essentially eating half a lunch while I decide on what to eat for lunch). I just choose from my options, and make it happen. All of these recipes are easy for me to pack up and take. If I'm traveling or on the go, it's super easy to get something similar at a restaurant. I know what I'm doing ahead of time for each meal, so I can enjoy my food and move on with my day. Same for my snacks:

SNACKS:

- Homemade turkey chili or vegetable soup (1 cup – like a big coffee mug's worth)

- Leftover roasted or sautéed vegetables from last night's dinner

- Half an avocado with pepper or red chili flakes (medium sized)

- Roast chicken thigh or 1/2 breast Birchermeusli or vanilla full-fat yogurt with walnuts

- A high quality bar (1/2 bar – nut-based, no grains, requires refrigeration)

- Baby carrots (3/4 Cup)

- Dark chocolate (one oz. or so, and maybe dipped in peanut butter!)

Dinners are Social Food meals for me several times each week – maybe one or two meals at restaurants or friends' houses and I eat high quality pasta (yep, I said pasta!) once or twice each week. Pizza, meatballs, and some sort of vegetable are our Thursday night staple. And often there's still a slice for my Saturday lunch. I definitely eat more Habit Food meals earlier in the week and save up Social Foods meals for special weeknight dinners out and weekends.

See? The strategy is awesome in its simplicity: from now on, like me and my clients, you will have a couple easy, delicious, nutritious items to choose from for each meal without using any brain power to do it. Take the time to really look at the ingredients of everything you eat most often, especially things that come from packages or jars. Make sure they are as clean as possible—no sugar syrups, no non-beneficial oils like corn or canola. Creating a strong foundation of nutritious foods upon which to rely each week is the key to making this work for you, both quickly and for the long haul.

Portioning How-To's

NUTRITION 101: MACRONUTRIENTS MAKE YOUR BODY GO

MACRONUTRIENT	PROVIDE ENERGY	GROWTH/ HEALING	REGULATE FUNCTIONS
Proteins	✔	✔	✔
Beneficial Fats	✔	✔	✔
Carbohydrates	✔		

Note: Vitamins/Minerals and Water are also essential for growth, healing, and regulation of body functions.

Your mom wasn't lying, vegetables are good for you. They should make up the largest portion of the total foods you eat in a day. If you find you're feeling hungry too soon after eating, make sure to get some satisfying beneficial fats and proteins. Lean proteins promote muscle growth and healing, but we don't need to overdo it as some popular diets suggest. We don't need to overdo anything. Use your common sense and listen to your body's needs.

I'm not going to dictate to the tablespoon how you structure your Habit Food meals. Please just know that it's important to have carbohydrates from non-starchy vegetables and fruit, lean proteins and beneficial fats. (There's a cheat sheet in Chapter 13 of this book if you're unclear about what they are). Whatever your portion is, eyeball half veggies and/or fruit and then mix or choose between protein and fat for the other half. If that's too much thinking, then just go even thirds of each macronutrient.

Bottom Line: If your Habit Food list is mostly fibrous, non-starchy veggies, quality proteins, and beneficial fats, you'll be golden.

If you are looking for ideas for what to eat at each meal, check out the hundreds of Habit Food recipes on my AND/life™ app. Check the back of the book for more sample menus and a list of non-starchy vegetables that provide nutrition, water and fiber without being too energy-dense like their starchy counterparts.

Social Foods

Habit Foods should make up about 80% percent of your meals, which leaves 20% for Social Meals. To put it simply, you get 7 or 8 Social Meals a week.

What does that mean exactly?

If your meal includes a Social Food, it becomes a Social Meal.

So, whether I eat two slices of pizza and nothing else for dinner or I have only once slice of pizza with a side salad, they're both counted the same – as Social Meals?

Yes. You'll get to your goals faster (and with greater nutrition in that meal) if you have one slice of pizza and a side salad. But if you're sticking to the strategy - 80% Habit Foods, suggested hand portions and eating schedule guidelines - you'll get to your goals nutritiously either way.

When new clients first come to me, so many of them struggle with the idea that your body isn't keeping score day by day—that one plate of fettuccini alfredo is going to sabotage your week (just be sure to follow portion guidelines). For the record, I struggled long and hard with this idea too! But your body is way more interested in what you do over a few days or a week. Strategizing your Habit Foods means enjoying your social life a lot! How's that for a super-easy, win-win, long-term, lean lifestyle strategy?

Desserts: Measure your pleasure

When dessert arrives at a Social Meal, start with the Rule of Awesome. Take one bite and, if the dessert is legitimately awesome, savor two more bites of it and be done. Put your fork down. (And do not use your fingers instead.)

The Three Bite Rule is essential to making it so you can always say yes to dessert and still achieve your fitness goals. Most likely, as your taste for sugar recalibrates after eating Habit Food ingredients 80% of the time, any more than three bites will be too sweet, too much and you'll self-regulate without issue. But here's a little extra motivation to keeping dessert to Three Bites:

Your body releases the pleasure hormone dopamine when you eat sweets. If you allow yourself too much at each sitting, you'll chronically

A WAY IN TO SUCCESS #6:
Skip the "Should Haves"

You're out at dinner with your friends, and you have two voices in your head: One says, "I really should have that raw kale salad…it's the responsible thing to do." The other says, "Ugh, are you kidding me? When they are famous for their Mac and Cheese?! Rachel's having a bacon cheeseburger, and you're going to have shredded paper?" My advice: Get the Mac and Cheese, eat an appropriate portion, and call it a day.

The number one goal in social situations is not to overeat. And if you've thought out your Habit Foods appropriately, it's OK to forgo the "should" foods for one meal. Follow the Rule of Awesome and have the thing you actually want.

You will be more successful at weight loss if you honor your desire for less nutritious foods and allow yourself to enjoy them from time to time. You'll find this permission is liberating. With Habit Foods as your nutritional foundation and a recalibrated stomach as your safety net, eating richer Social Foods will cost you nothing in the long run.

have too much dopamine floating around and your body will remove some of your dopamine sensors. This means you will need more bites of dessert to get the same level of pleasure you used to get from just a few bites.

As your tastes recalibrate with sugar significantly lessened by this food strategy, your brain will reset to where you'll get a lot of dopamine bang from your dessert right at the first few bites. Maintain that delicate balance by applying the Rule of Awesome plus the Three Bite Rule and you'll start to be one of "those people" who seem to be able to eat anything and still be in great shape.

Caloric Drinks

If flab won't seem to budge or you seem to be at a permanent plateau despite your best efforts with food and exercise, calories in the beverages you drink might be the culprit. Juices, blended coffee drinks, smoothies made with juice (or sweetened nondairy milks), sweetened teas, and alcoholic beverages all inject boatloads of calories into your diet that aren't needed for energy – your got that covered with food. And caloric beverages can be a double whammy because they tend to deliver energy from sugar carbs but without insulin-moderating fiber, protein or fat. This means they might be slowing down your metabolism at the same time you're taking in more calories than you actually need at the moment.

THE WAY IN GUIDELINES FOR HYDRATION

Each day aim for:

- 8-10 glasses of water

- 2 or fewer caloric drinks

- 80% total non-caloric drinks

So here's the math:

- 6 glasses of water, 2 glasses unsweetened tea, one small latte, one glass of wine = 80%

- 9 glasses of water, 2 coffees with splash of milk (doesn't count as caloric), 2 cocktails = 83%

So again, like with Habit and Social foods, this is about making advantageous choices at least 80% of the time and allowing yourself social choices each day, if you want. 8oz is your portion.

I hope I don't need to tell you that for "cocktails," I mean small, relatively simple ones – liquor and a mixer. Big dessert drinks - strawberry margaritas, peach daquiri's, pina coladas - are the equivalent of cake. You cannot drink a whole one every day. You could have a few sips, like I suggest with bites of dessert as a social food, but who's really going to do that? The answer is, don't order dessert drinks unless you plan to count it as two portions.

Nutrition Tips to Keep in Mind

As you start on this journey, focus on the big ideas. Habit Foods are the ones in the "tree." Since portion control and schedule are the most important part of this plan, it doesn't have to be any more complicated than that.

With that said, as you move forward on your journey to health, you want to make the best food choices possible. So, once you are on the right track, begin to think about the following tips for making the best food choices.

Please note: I do not want you to memorize these guidelines the day you get started! Bookmark this page and come back when you're ready to take your plan to the next level.

Nutrition best hints and tips:

Once you start making Habit Food lists, come back to this page occasionally for ideas of how to improve your go-to's even more!

- **Choose lots of colors.** Deep green foods should be your foundation, but pick a variety of colorful fruits and veggies.

- **Be carb-conscious.** We need carbs. But the ones we need most of are non-starchy vegetable and fruits. If you find you're not losing the weight you want but you're eating on plan, filling up on calorie-dense starchy veggies, grains and beans may be the culprit. As a general rule, limit starchy carbs, grains and beans to one-hand portions at a time, and no more than two servings per day.

- **Breakfast cereals have never helped someone lose weight.** To be clear, I have zero quality science to back me on this. But for 25 years, my observation is that people who start their day with cereal—even clean, lower calorie kinds—never do as well as my clients who start with a quality protein/fat combo. No added sugar, whole-grain cereal is not off limits, but please try other options first to get yourself going. Maybe then reintroduce cereal once you're losing weight to see if it affects you in a negative way.

- **Real food goes bad.** Limited Habit Foods can be packaged as long as they are as clean and simple as possible. Opt for foods that require refrigeration and/or aren't designed to last forever. Frozen veggies don't have the sodium and preservatives found in canned foods. Beware of the sodium in canned beans – rinse them well. Same for tomato products – buy the best quality and lowest in sodium you can find.

- **Get an insurance policy for high-carb foods.** Findings from a Tufts University study published in on September 7, 2016 in the American Journal of Clinical Nutrition shows that blood sugar spikes from carbs not only vary by person, but also for each person by day. In other words, tomorrow you may be better at digesting a banana eaten on its own than you are today.

WHAT? I know. And just like that, we're back to the idea that you're not a machine.

Yes, it would be great if we could all break ourselves down to simple spreadsheet-worthy math and graph our way to shrinking. But alas, we are human and therefore we must strategize. And the best strategy to temper blood sugar spikes that may occur when you eat high-glycemic foods (like bread, pasta, and potatoes) is to always eat a quality protein with them (lean meat or nuts). If that's not available, then a good fat.

- **Follow the Two Fat Rule.** Fats are good for us, but we still need to eat them in moderation. Limit your fats at each setting to just two—so if you have a salad with avocado and olive oil-based dressing, don't add cheese too. If you have a cheese omelet cooked in butter or oil, opt for veggies rather than breakfast meats.

- **Choose better condiments.** Condiments and seasonings are fine—and some are great. Hot sauces and cinnamon have natural metabolism boosters (though minimal), and vinegar products, especially fermented ones, help digestion. Ketchup, however, and most dressings have tons of sugar, additives, and texturizers (blech). Consider these Social Foods or buy options that are all-natural.

- **Hydrate between meals, not while you eat**. You may have heard that you should drink water before you eat in order to eat less, but all that does is stretch out your stomach (the opposite of our goal) and dilute your digestive enzymes. Absolutely drink 8 to 10 glasses of water a day. But don't do it while you are eating. Drink a comfortable amount to wash down your food but remember what I always say: too much, even of a good thing, is still too much.

- **Be aware of the sugar in milk substitutes.** When using plant-based milks, opt for ones with the lowest possible sugar, some fiber and insulin-curbing protein and/or fat.

- **Eat your calories, don't drink them.** Opt for real food instead of icey, blended coffee concoctions, pressed juices that costs as much as liquid gold or "super healthy" green smoothies (unless they're super low in sugar and contain protein – and no, you don't need 54g of it in one meal).

A Final Word

A lot of people don't believe me at first, but I have a catalog of success stories to back this up, and I promise you: by eating Habit Foods for most of your meals, your taste buds will change! As days and weeks go by, you will naturally start to shy away from, and eventually reject, Low Value Social Foods. You'll end up eating cleaner foods almost all the time by choice, not to be "good" – and that's the beginning of true food freedom.

Bon Appetit!

10

LIFE ISN'T A MEDAL EVENT, SO STOP TRAINING FOR THE OLYMPICS™

BY THIS POINT IN THE BOOK, after I've made a case that the most important components of good health are when, how much, and what you *eat*, you may be thinking, *wait, isn't this lady a fitness trainer?*

The answer is, yes, the foundation of my expertise is in exercise. Creating effective and engaging workouts has been my bread and butter for over 25 years. I've spent tens of thousands of hours on the subject of exercise and have helped hundreds of people elevate themselves. And all of this experience has led me to a crucial conclusion: exercise and weight loss don't always go hand-in-hand.

Have you ever had one of those New Year's where you get super fired-up about your resolution to work out? Of course, you have! You outfit yourself in superhero–worthy tech-fabric clothing, the latest cross-training shoes that weigh less than a gerbil and your new personal monitoring gizmo that helps make sure you hit your "goal" numbers... And you start waking up early and maybe you sign yourself up for a marathon or get a membership at the "nicer" gym in town or make a point to book spinning class weeks ahead, so you can get a bike in front... Point is: you're motivated, you're dedicated, you're following through... but your scale doesn't budge. So, what's the deal? Why haven't you "run your ass off" yet?

It seems like simple math – take in fewer calories than you need and burn more than you have available, so your body will turn to fat for fuel and you'll lose weight. But this simple math doesn't take into account the human factors that affect weight like hormones, hydration, rest and, importantly, how exercise type and intensity affects how we *feel* and how we *eat*. Also, sorry to be the spoiler, but both your calorie counting wearable and the elliptical machine at the gym estimate calorie burn based on general factors about you and outdated heart rate to calorie burn estimation formulas set against general human averages. You might be burning way fewer calories than your gadget reports.

Exercise intensity and duration are crucial factors. Too much is too much and it's crucial to figure out where that line is for you – the line where your workouts affect your need for food in a way that makes weight loss slow or stagnant. Some people thrive with high intensity workouts while others feel really off if they burn out too much glycogen (muscle sugar), leaving them feeling funny and very depleted. (As strong and physically capable as I am, BTW, I'm actually one of those people.) For many of you, we need to amp up your exercise for sure, but like food, it's not a one-size-fits-all prescription. You need to find the right balance, so your amped-up exercise program doesn't end up working against you by making you need to eat even more to try to feel "right" or ravenous from burning up so many calories so quickly.

Additionally, because you're overtired from workouts that are too much, your hunger hormones go into overdrive. You start eating a few bites extra at every meal or just start eating so fast because you feel ravenous that you routinely take in more calories than you need before your brain can catch up and let you know you're satisfied.

And all that extra food is making you feel bloated. So, what do you do? Take an extra-long spinning class the next day to try to feel less gross. Which then just makes you super hungry again. But that's OK, you think, because your gizmo said you burned more calories than you ate all last week. Plus, you're doing what a champ does – you're pushing and pushing, harder than the other guy so you can turn your jelly-arms into ice sculptures and your keg-abs into a six-pack.

And you're counting your "macros" and your "micros"... and yes, the scales's going up - but that's OK you tell yourself, because it's "lean muscle tissue" you're developing! And pretty soon that muscle is going to be meta-bolically advantageous – because you'll burn more just "existing" than you did before! Which makes you think maybe you should be eating more protein so you can build even more muscle so your metabolism will go even faster cause that's what it says on the internet so it must be right. And never eat bread! Or a banana! And once you do all those things, it's all going to come together! You'll finally be a metabolic wonder with all that lean muscle tissue you built via Herculean workouts and buckets of protein and principled avoidance of the C-word (carbs)… and your arms will be ripped, and your abs will chiseled and you'll fit into those jeans from six years ago and you'll be happy!!!!!!!!

But then it doesn't all come together, and you're exhausted, and you actu-ally need to buy bigger jeans and don't even get you started on your arms as they seem to be getting bigger and bigger but no less doughy and you're anything but happy.

And if you are the small percentage of people I've seen who (miraculously) do get to the body of their dreams with Navy Seal-worthy workouts, guess what happens when life intervenes and they can't keep up the exercise regimen? In the event you haven't personally experienced this, I'll tell you: with stomachs now adapted to massive portions of food and that don't care that they're not box jumping their way to fabulous anymore, they gain the weight right back. The point of "satisfied" for your stomach after an uber-heavy workout/lots and lots of food approach will now be way more calories than you need if you're not working out for an hour and half plus standing most of the day. And you will watch yourself grow larger again. Except for your smile, which is the only thing you'll see shrink until you get a better strategy.

So, if working out isn't how we lose weight, what's the point?

I'm glad you asked. Unless you are a professional athlete or are working to achieve a specific physical goal like running a marathon or competing in a Spartan race, let's realign the purpose of exercise once and for all:

- Increase the overall health and efficiency of your heart and lungs

- Achieve and maintain a healthy level of body fat

- Develop strong, toned muscles to live more freely and move with confidence

- Improve posture that allows you to live pain-free

- Increase flexibility to heal and prevent joint and back pain

- Look awesome in pictures, at reunions, and when your run into your ex

Countless women and men have come to me upset that they gained weight after committing to use their month-long unlimited pass to a boutique spinning studio or ended up bigger and with even less definition after taking a month of aggressive classes "guaranteed" to be muscle-chiseling and fat-blasting.

Exercise is a tool. How you use it determines how much you benefit from it. If you want to run a marathon, do it! Train until those 26.2 miles seem less daunting, knowing that you may not lose any weight in the process. If you want to compete in extreme sports, then by all means, join your local gym's ninja warrior program.

The goals of my exercise program are:

- **Look great and feel strong**

- **Develop confidence and mental clarity**

- **Support weight loss**

- **End up with a toned, lean physique that's easy to maintain**

If these goals are your goals, you don't need extreme workouts—you need a strategy.

Before I tell my clients *how* to exercise, I talk to them about *why* they need to exercise. And so far, not one person has come in and said, "to win a pull-up contest" or "to perform at the level of a professional athlete." Instead, everyone wants the same thing: ladies want to look long and strong, guys want to look ripped and tall, and everyone wants to feel lean, energetic and free of chronic aches and pains.

Surprisingly, the prescription is similar (although the resistance required varies widely from person to person and between women and men). The best, most time-efficient way to achieve that fit physique is to alternate between moderate cardio (fast-paced walking or on equipment) and what I call "Resistance Cardio" sessions, around 20 minutes a pop with longer and higher intensity workouts thrown in a few times each week as you work towards your goal.

During the Six Week Shape-Up program, we will push the duration of some workouts all the way to 40-60 minutes to hasten development of strength, stamina and fat loss. The physical conditioning achieved during this program will allow you to maximize shorter workouts as you continue on your own. Beyond these six weeks, 20-30 minutes of daily heart-rate up exercise (and yes, walking is fine for some of those days) coupled with 60 minutes of daily standing is the lifestyle as far as exercise is concerned. Occasional longer workouts are great, but not if they are unsustainable as a lifestyle and make you need to eat more.

For some readers, a 20-40-minute workout is 20-40 minutes more than they have ever done regularly. Never fear - this plan is going to build up slowly, giving your body the space and time it needs to change for good. Soon, getting your heart rate up will be integrated into your daily schedule in a way that is totally manageable.

For my exercise-junkies, it's a drastic cut-back and I know how you feel. I was terrified when I took the flying leap 9 years ago to experiment on myself with my theories before foisting them on my clients. Please hear me when I promise you that you aren't going to get anywhere by overtraining. Moderate exercise and an active lifestyle will take you a lot further toward your goals than grueling workouts followed by sitting all day. We're going to find a lifestyle that is still challenging, but even more sustainable, and that doesn't require you to spend hours every day at the gym. Because don't you have better things to do?

So, here's what the plan looks like:

PHASE 1 – FOUNDATION (weeks 1-2): You will start at a moderate baseline of daily exercise and activity, the foundation for your new, more dynamic lifestyle. Your focus will be on committing to your 20 minutes of getting your heart rate up – even if all you can fit on some days is walking. Also, you'll start standing a total of 60 extra minutes each day.

PHASE 2 - STRENGTH & STAMINA (weeks 3-4): Now that you are used to daily activity (or adjusted to dialed-down moderate activity for my former sweat-a-holics), we will work on ramping both your strength and stamina by adding resistance work to almost every session. The goal is to maximize your workout time by combining cardio with muscle development while developing baseline strength and stamina.

PHASE 3 – RAMP UP (weeks 5-6): These two weeks will show you how to push yourself so that you are able to continue making progress on your own and avoid plateaus. We will incorporate high-intensity intervals into your resistance work to fast-track the strengthening of your heart and lungs, increase your overall exercise capacity and, most importantly, create metabolism-boosting afterburn.

Before we get into the nitty-gritty of this plan, it's important to know the thought behind it.

WALK AWAY (FROM FLAB)

Getting lean isn't a sprint; it's a walk. Once again, I'm going to risk putting myself out of business to tell you that walking—simple, one foot in front of the other—is the key to being fit for life.

Now, is walking going to give you Instagram-worthy abs? No. That will come later. But as a core activity, walking is the best and easiest way to make sure you're active every day.

Starting with week one on the Six Week Shape Up (and for the rest of your life on The Way In lifestyle), your bare minimum daily exercise goal is to walk at least 20 minutes. That's 10 minutes in one direction and 10 minutes back at a decent clip. If you don't feel like strolling around outside or on a treadmill, you can substitute a piece of cardio equipment at the gym such as an elliptical, upright bike or stair climber for the treadmill or a walk outside. The point here is to consistently put in a moderate amount of physical activity for 20 consecutive minutes every day.

I know you are busy. I know it's hard to find time for ourselves. But a 20-minute walk? That's doable. Do you have a call you need to make? Take your phone and head outside (just please be sure to pay attention as you cross the street!) Are you catching up on your favorite show? Watch it on the treadmill, or even better, the stair climber. Do you check Facebook or Twitter? Do it while you walk. While you're "liking" your friends' posts, show yourself some actual love by moving around.

STAND UP FOR YOURSELF

We waste—er, *spend*—so much time every day sitting. And it turns out this may be worse for us than we thought.

In recent years we've learned that sitting all day is not only a missed opportunity to move—it's actively destructive to our health. According to findings reported by the American Heart Association (Circulation, August 16, 2016), even an hour a day of vigorous physical activity (meaning all-out, sweat-pouring, heart-pumping exercise) doesn't cancel out the negative impact of spending the rest of the day on your backside. Further, the AHA determined that sitting most of the day increases the risk of cardiovascular disease and diabetes, *even among people who exercise regularly.* Yikes!

For some of our daily tasks, we have no choice but to nestle into our chairs—perhaps someday a standing-car will be invented, but for now, we're stuck on our butts. A lot of our daily activities, however, could be mobile or at least standing. Reading books and the newspaper, looking at social media, studying, watching TV—every minute you choose to stand rather than sit, you're getting your blood pumping, relieving your spine and hip muscles of pressure, and giving yourself a metabolic booster shot for the rest of your day. My kitchen counter has become my best friend – I set up my laptop and work there half the day at least. When I host guests, I stand behind that counter as much of the time as possible – certainly through cocktails and after dinner.

From now on, you're going to stand more every day, starting with 60 extra minutes and working your way up to 90. It might sound like a lot, but it isn't; it's just 10 minutes here, 20 minutes there. You don't have to force this—start small by agreeing to stand every time you have to make a call. Switch from sitting while you fold laundry to standing. It's easy, and you don't have to adjust your schedule at all. Eventually, you'll prefer the feeling of your body being at its full length, stretching out and moving around, instead of slumping into a chair.

REST

A full night of sleep – whatever that means for you - is one of your most critical **daily habits**, which is why you need a strategy! Maybe that means turning off your screens or unwinding with meditation. Perhaps it's setting an alarm to get into bed. Whatever you need to do, make sure to get a full night's rest. They don't call it "beauty sleep" for nothing!

RESISTANCE CARDIO

Once walking and regular movement are a firm part of your routine, we will incorporate what I call Resistance Cardio sessions. These are functional, total body workouts designed to accomplish two goals with the shortest time commitment:

- TONE MUSCLES: Resistance uses either equipment or the weight of your own body to build lean muscle tissue. And thoughtfully developed muscle will improve your metabolism, helping to melt layers of flab faster. Evenly developed muscle also improves your alignment, alleviating pain... and, yes, looks great too.

- STRENGTHEN YOUR HEART AND LUNGS: Cardiovascular exercise elevates your heart rate. Clinically, cardio improves your "VO2 Max," - the volume of oxygen your heart can transport with every pump. You will come to recognize improvement in VO2 Max as, "Hey, I just climbed up that flight of stairs and I'm not out of breath."

The key to any resistance exercise program is to be sure to work your entire body evenly and 3-5 times per week once you build up some stamina and strength. If you're not super well-versed in anatomy and physiology as they relate to exercise, never fear: I've created a huge variety of great classes on my AND/life™ app. You can also use the app to create balanced custom workouts based on your personal preferences.

What you won't find as a part of this program or on the AND/life™ app is "leg day" or "back day." That's the protocol for a traditional body-building approach where the goal is big muscles and the way they look is more important than how they perform. This is an entirely different philosophy with specific nutritional requirements to achieve extreme muscle hypertrophy (mass) rather than weight loss and a toned, physique.

THE WAY IN TO SUCCESS:
To get the weight off, get your sleep on!

For obvious reasons, better sleep means better weight loss. Rest ensures you have the energy to move when you want, helps you make better decisions, and allows your body to burn more calories when you're inactive. But the amount of sleep you get doesn't just affect whether or not you'll be able to lose weight, it also decides the kind of weight you will lose.

A study published in the Annals of Internal Medicine (*Insufficient Sleep Undermines Dietary Efforts to Reduce Adiposity*; October 5, 2010) showed that dieters who slept eight hours per night lost weight mostly from fat (yay!), while more than half of the pounds dropped by dieters who slept only five hours each night came from muscle (boo!).

Further, the study showed that after just two weeks of not getting enough sleep, your body starts producing more ghrelin—the hunger hormone—and less leptin—the "stop eating, I'm full" hormone. In other words, sleep deprivation makes you think you're hungry when you're not and inhibits your ability to know when you're full. Push your bedtime too late and run the risk of sabotaging your health journey.

I started my career with a traditional strength training approach and didn't like the result on me or any of my clients – especially because I hadn't yet developed this winning approach to food. What I found over time is that diversified exercise delivers better results and overall fitness. During the Six Week Shape-Up, you will try three types of resistance workouts: strength training with weights, Pilates or yoga. You will also try different types of cardio and high-intensity interval training. Use your LIFEtracker form to keep track of your workouts each week and how they made you feel so that we can figure out which combinations of workouts and food work best for your body.

HIGH-INTENSITY INTERVAL TRAINING

High-Intensity Interval Training (HIIT) improves your cardiovascular health, ramps up your overall fitness level, and (here's the part you care about) boosts your metabolism to burn fat throughout the day even after your workout. This methodology is characterized by bouts of all-out effort lasting from :30 seconds to 2 minutes, followed by active rest (gentle movement) until your heart rate drops to just a bit above normal before proceeding again.

At first, getting your heart rate to come down may take up to two (or more) minutes until your overall fitness improves. In fact, how quickly your heart rate returns to normal is one of the easiest ways trainers can gauge client progress - the more fit people are, the faster their heart rates return to normal. It's essential to wait for this critical moment (i.e., you can breathe and speak easily) before you go again into another interval. It's the "0-60" demand on your heart and lungs that makes this type of work so effective at getting your body to improve rapidly. In short, HIIT training is a fitness "fast track" you definitely want to get on.

That said, a word of caution is in order: precisely because HIIT is so effective at burning fat and ramping up fitness, people do too much, too often and for too long, which then actually lessens the impact. They take hour long classes with instructors who encourage everyone to work at the same pace (super-hard) and without allowing enough time for individual heart rates to have returned to a low enough place for the work to be truly effective. People feel depleted – because they are - which makes them turn to food and caloric sports drinks to feel normal again, essentially putting back into their system all the stored calories (flab) they hoped to mobilize off their bodies.

Always leave a day between workouts that include HIIT training, so your body has adequate time to heal and restore itself. Never risk injury in the name of burning calories. Remember, this is a long-haul game of burning fat off your body (yes, as fast as possible!) and that exercise is the compliment to the food strategy, not the other way around. Overdoing it won't help and can slow your progress by driving you straight into a plateau or creating issues like tendonitis or muscle strains that will take the tool of exercise away from you.

How do we measure "high intensity"? You could track your heart rate, but as with our approach to food, my experience has shown me the value of being less reliant on mathematical data, and more in-tune to your body's signs and signals. If you are already fit and looking to motivate yourself by trying to "better your best," data can help you set personal benchmarks to exceed. But as you're learning how your body best operates, I prefer the no-gadget approach, using the classic Rate of Perceived Exertion, or the RPE scale.

MODIFIED RATE OF PERCEIVED EXERTION CHART

RPE	DESCRIPTION
0-1 No effort	You're watching TV wondering what to get for a snack during the next commercial break.
2-3 Light effort	You're meandering through a meadow on a sunny day, gazing up to see if the clouds overhead look more like bunnies or dragons.
4-5 Medium effort	After overhearing a lady say Ryan Gosling was at the Apple Store, you're glowing a bit as you hustle across the mall while trying not to seem like a crazy person.
6-7 Medium-hard effort	You are flat out sweating and short of breath as you race to catch the taxi where you just left your cell phone.
8-9 Hard effort	Sweating buckets, you can't talk at all as you sprint through the airport to make your plane home for Thanksgiving dinner.
10	Yep, that's a lion chasing you.

Workout intensity during your Six Week Shape-Up will vary by type of exercise:

- Walks or moderate cardio: 4-5 RPE

- Resistance work (weights, Pilates, yoga): 5-6 RPE

- HIIT (High Intensity Interval Training): 8-9 RPE for :30 sec–2 min
  4 RPE active rest target

Your LIFEtracker worksheets will help you keep notes on which workouts left you feeling strong, energized and inspired to do it again. Those are the ones you will lean on most as you continue with the lifestyle.

Speaking of which, next up, we will put all the strategies together - food, hydration, exercise and standing - for the full six-week plan and the start of your new lifestyle!

THE WAY IN LIFESTYLE:
DAILY GOALS AT A GLANCE

 Food: schedule, portions, 80% Habit Foods

 Hydration: 80% non-caloric drinks each week, at least 8-10 glasses each day

 Exercise: 20 minutes per day

 Standing: 60 minutes per day to start, working your way up to at least 90 minutes

11

THE SIX WEEK SHAPE-UP

IT'S TIME TO DIVE INTO THE SIX WEEK SHAPE-UP! This fast-paced program has been designed to systematically create habits that:

·   Rev your metabolism

·   Shrink your stomach

·   Change your taste away from sugary, salty, and greasy foods

·   Increase your strength and stamina

·   Incorporate exercise and daily movement into your life

The Six Week Shape-Up is not the lifestyle you will lead once you complete the program. It is the *learning process* for your mind and body - The Way In - to your new long-term, fitness lifestyle.

The Way In lifestyle you will lead after this program is simpler than what you will be asked to do in the Shape-Up. The basic pillars of The Way In lifestyle are four, doable daily goals:

·   Eat 80% Habit Food Meals and 20% Social Food Meals

·   Drink 80% non-caloric beverages total, aiming for 8-10 glasses of water daily

·   Exercise (get your heart rate up) 20 minutes every day

·   Stand at least 60 minutes every day

By completing the progress analysis worksheets at the end of the program, you will be able to see how closely you need to adhere to these pillars to continue "shaping-up" and stay that way. For example, some people can get away with more Social Foods than they think. Some people need to have even fewer caloric drinks. Some people do better with fewer high intensity workouts. Some people need that extra boost more often. The important thing is to find out what YOU need so you can keep progressing in a way that is totally doable!

HABIT FOOD WORKSHEETS

The first thing you'll find in this chapter are your Habit Food Worksheets. Each week, you'll be guided to come up with new food ideas you find compelling and, most importantly, easy to make. At the end of the six weeks, these pages will be filled with solid lists of go-to foods for each meal – your "rotation." Thanks to these lists, never again will you say, "I don't know what to eat." And not only that, once you complete your Progress Analysis, you'll have figured out which amongst these food ideas can be counted on to make you feel your absolute best!

WEEK-BY-WEEK PROGRAM

After your Habit Food Worksheets, you'll find the Six Week Shape-Up program, outlined week-by-week. After each week's goals are explained, they are listed for you on a comprehensive LIFEtracker form, so you can track your choices and achievements simply by checking off hand portions, drinks and boxes labeled for workouts. Also, there is space at the bottom to make note of foods or workouts that feel particularly great (or not so great). You'll get the most value from the program by being sure to note not only results, but how food and workouts made you *feel*.

PROGRESS ANALYSIS

After the final week of the Shape-Up, you'll find two progress analysis work-sheets: your Fitness Lifestyle Formula and your Rapid Reset Formula. This is where all your choices and results come together to create your truly effective, personal program. You will discover what you can "get away with" in terms of Social Foods and caloric drinks and keep moving toward your goals. You will also learn which of your workouts are most effective and resonate on a strong emotional level so that you look forward to continuing with daily exercise. Lastly, you will zero in on your "best of the best" – the foods and workouts which delivered results the fastest - to uncover your Rapid Reset Formula for times when you need a quick boost.

I can't wait to start this journey with you, so let's get going!

NOTES

HABIT FOODS *worksheet*

List your new Go-To Meal ideas here. Achieve success each week by alternating between only two or three choices for each meal.

breakfast

Go-To Option 1: _____ Go-To for Week(s) 1 2 3 4 5 6 *(circle)*

Go-To Option 2: _____ Go-To for Week(s) 1 2 3 4 5 6 *(circle)*

Go-To Option 3: _____ Go-To for Week(s) 1 2 3 4 5 6 *(circle)*

Go-To Option 4: _____ Go-To for Week(s) 1 2 3 4 5 6 *(circle)*

Best Habit Food Go-To 1: _____ Go-To for Week(s) 1 2 3 4 5 6 *(circle)*

Best Habit Food Go-To 2: _____ Go-To for Week(s) 1 2 3 4 5 6 *(circle)*

Other 1: _____ Go-To for Week(s) 1 2 3 4 5 6 *(circle)*

Other 2: _____ Go-To for Week(s) 1 2 3 4 5 6 *(circle)*

mid-morning snack

Go-To Option 1: _____ Go-To for Week(s) 1 2 3 4 5 6 *(circle)*

Go-To Option 2: _____ Go-To for Week(s) 1 2 3 4 5 6 *(circle)*

Go-To Option 3: _____ Go-To for Week(s) 1 2 3 4 5 6 *(circle)*

Best Habit Food Go-To 1: _____ Go-To for Week(s) 1 2 3 4 5 6 *(circle)*

Other 1: _____ Go-To for Week(s) 1 2 3 4 5 6 *(circle)*

Other 2: _____ Go-To for Week(s) 1 2 3 4 5 6 *(circle)*

Breakfast Motivation:

When in doubt (or a super rush), make a two-hand portion of a single Go-To Meal option and divide between breakfast and your mid-morning snack. It doesn't get easier than that!

NOTES

HABIT FOODS *worksheet*

List your new Go-To Meal ideas here. Achieve success each week by alternating between only two or three choices for each meal.

lunch

Go-To Option 1: _____ Go-To for Week(s) 1 2 3 4 5 6 *(circle)*

Go-To Option 2: _____ Go-To for Week(s) 1 2 3 4 5 6 *(circle)*

Go-To Option 3: _____ Go-To for Week(s) 1 2 3 4 5 6 *(circle)*

Go-To Option 4: _____ Go-To for Week(s) 1 2 3 4 5 6 *(circle)*

Best Habit Food Go-To 1: _____ Go-To for Week(s) 1 2 3 4 5 6 *(circle)*

Best Habit Food Go-To 2: _____ Go-To for Week(s) 1 2 3 4 5 6 *(circle)*

Other 1: _____ Go-To for Week(s) 1 2 3 4 5 6 *(circle)*

Other 2: _____ Go-To for Week(s) 1 2 3 4 5 6 *(circle)*

afternoon snack

Go-To Option 1: _____ Go-To for Week(s) 1 2 3 4 5 6 *(circle)*

Go-To Option 2: _____ Go-To for Week(s) 1 2 3 4 5 6 *(circle)*

Best Habit Food Go-To 1: _____ Go-To for Week(s) 1 2 3 4 5 6 *(circle)*

Best Habit Food Go-To 2: _____ Go-To for Week(s) 1 2 3 4 5 6 *(circle)*

Other 1: _____ Go-To for Week(s) 1 2 3 4 5 6 *(circle)*

Other 2: _____ Go-To for Week(s) 1 2 3 4 5 6 *(circle)*

❗ Lunch Motivation:

Lose weight faster and keep it off by sticking to your weekly Habit Food plan no matter where you are. Treat quick, grab-and-go meals out as if you were the cook: skip the menu and order as closely as possible to the Go-To Meal you would have made yourself.

NOTES

HABIT FOODS *worksheet*

List your new Go-To Meal ideas here. Achieve success each week by alternating between only two or three choices for each meal.

dinner

Go-To Option 1: _____ Go-To for Week(s) 1 2 3 4 5 6 *(circle)*

Go-To Option 2: _____ Go-To for Week(s) 1 2 3 4 5 6 *(circle)*

Go-To Option 3: _____ Go-To for Week(s) 1 2 3 4 5 6 *(circle)*

Go-To Option 4: _____ Go-To for Week(s) 1 2 3 4 5 6 *(circle)*

Go-To Option 5: _____ Go-To for Week(s) 1 2 3 4 5 6 *(circle)*

Go-To Option 6: _____ Go-To for Week(s) 1 2 3 4 5 6 *(circle)*

Best Habit Food Go-To 1: _____ Go-To for Week(s) 1 2 3 4 5 6 *(circle)*

Best Habit Food Go-To 2: _____ Go-To for Week(s) 1 2 3 4 5 6 *(circle)*

Best Habit Food Go-To 3: _____ Go-To for Week(s) 1 2 3 4 5 6 *(circle)*

Best Habit Food Go-To 4: _____ Go-To for Week(s) 1 2 3 4 5 6 *(circle)*

Other 1: _____ Go-To for Week(s) 1 2 3 4 5 6 *(circle)*

Other 2: _____ Go-To for Week(s) 1 2 3 4 5 6 *(circle)*

evening snack

Go-To Option 1: _____ Go-To for Week(s) 1 2 3 4 5 6 *(circle)*

Go-To Option 2: _____ Go-To for Week(s) 1 2 3 4 5 6 *(circle)*

Go-To Option 3: _____ Go-To for Week(s) 1 2 3 4 5 6 *(circle)*

Best Habit Food Go-To 1: _____ Go-To for Week(s) 1 2 3 4 5 6 *(circle)*

Other 1: _____ Go-To for Week(s) 1 2 3 4 5 6 *(circle)*

Other 2: _____ Go-To for Week(s) 1 2 3 4 5 6 *(circle)*

★ Dinner Motivation:

Whether eating Habit Foods or Social Foods, live by the Rule of Awesome: bring each day to a close with beautiful food that excites your senses and lifts your soul.

SIX WEEK SHAPE-UP: WEEK ONE

THE BIG PICTURE

This week we will tackle two priorities: we will begin by calibrating your stomach and then we will introduce Habit Foods.

   During Days 1-3, eat any foods you want. No kidding. Your only focus for the first three days of this program is to get your food portions and eating schedule in gear according to guidelines.

   During days 4-7, you will eat Habit Foods only. Use days 1-3 to prepare: keep going with the Habit Foods page you started, completing your first rotation of Habit Food meals and shopping for any new foods you need! Remember that if the food you already eat fits Habit Food criteria, leave it alone for now. Changing as few recipes as possible will increase your likelihood for success. For foods and recipes that don't make the cut, the AND/life™ app is full of great ideas.

   Starting on Day 4, you will also begin the drinks strategy – which can sometimes be more challenging for people than the food. Because beverages can be one of the biggest hidden spoilers to weight loss efforts, we will start with 90% non-caloric drinks per week – that means one 8 oz. caloric drink per day. Don't worry—this is not forever! But for right now, help yourself get to your best self as fast as possible by strategizing your caloric drinks. (Don't worry. A splash of milk in your coffee doesn't count as your caloric drink.)

For activity, the first two weeks of the program are about building baseline strength and stamina by getting your heart rate up for 20 minutes each day, and creating an active lifestyle that includes consistent, moderate workouts and habitual standing – daily activity that burns stored energy without making you need to eat more. For some people, it'll take a week or two to make this time a "want-to" and "need-to" rather than a "have-to." For others who are used to working out an hour at a pop, please take the flying leap and dial it back to 20 mins each day just for this week and simply stand, walk and be "up-and-about" more.

Note your choices and how you feel this week on your Week One LIFEtracker Page. Even if it's just the quickest scribble at the end of each day to recap, do it. Your notes will be crucial to unlocking your personal fitness formula by the end of the next six weeks.

FOOD

Days 1-3: Calibration – Follow portion and schedule guidelines to begin systematically "shrinking" your stomach so you are naturally, honestly full with less food at each meal or snack time. Don't worry about *what* you eat. Spend three days learning *how* to eat.

- Follow portion guidelines and eat every 2 to 4 hours starting within one hour of waking. This will add up to 5-6 meals per day.

- Complete your first list of Habit Foods to include:

  - 2 breakfast

  - 2 lunch options

  - 4 snack options

  - 4 dinner options

- Make sure to be aware of Limited Habit Foods and have only 2 or less per day for each kind.

Days 4-7: First Habit Foods – Integrate Best and Limited Habit Foods into at least 5 meals per day. One meal per day can (and should) include Social Foods.

- Begin alternating the food ideas you've chosen for breakfasts, lunches and snacks.

- Dinner may change nightly and very well end up being a Social Meal – that's fine.

- Include Social Foods up to four times. For example, if you order an all Habit Food salad at a restaurant, but then eat some of your friend's fries, record that in your LIFEtracker page as a social meal.

- Eat only real food. No chips or low value grazing foods - not even "healthy" ones. Eat foods lower in sugar and sodium whenever possible, even in Social Foods.

Drinks: Weight Loss Strategy – 8-10 8 oz. non-caloric, beneficial beverages each day, plus no more than one 8 oz. caloric drink per day.

EXERCISE

- Four days this week, do 20-30 mins of brisk walking or other moderate cardio.

- Do three 20-minute workouts this week that include resistance (i.e., weights, yoga, Pilates). You can either do resistance work for all 20 minutes or split the time into 10 minutes resistance plus 10 minutes of cardio.

- Record your workout time and notes on your LIFEtracker page.

STANDING

- Stand an extra 60 mins each day (total, does not have to be consecutive).

LEARN

Sugar & Sodium

Habit Foods are naturally lower in sugar and sodium, but you still may be getting more than is ideal. Don't worry about the naturally-occurring sugar and sodium in fruits and veggies. But please do start checking out labels of your condiments, dairy foods, yogurt or plant-based yogurt substitutes and all beverages. Also, get a sense of the sugar and sodium in any frozen proteins you eat often (i.e. organic turkey meatballs), wine or whatever cocktails you commonly order when out.

Remember, you don't need to cut out these foods. The knowledge is to help you strategize so on days when you know you'll be having foods higher in sodium or sugar (i.e., you know you're going out to dinner), eat the least sugary or salty Habit Foods options you have for other meals to counterbalance.

Sodium: stay under a ½ tsp per day of sodium (1150mg)

Sugar: stay under 14 tsp per day of added sugar (59g)

Portions by Sight

Take some time to find out what drink sizes look like in your own glasses. If you can recognize an 8 oz. serving in every glass you own, not only will you be more likely to stick with fitness-friendly portions, you may very well drop 5-10 unwanted pounds this year from this single adjustment alone.

NOTES

_____

_____

_____

_____

LIFE*tracker*

WEEK 1

Start Weight [ ] End Weight [ ] Change In Weight [ ] Goal = 2lbs.

Habit Food Meals	Way In Portion Guide	Mon.	Tues.	Wed.	Thurs.	Fri.	Sat.	Sun.	Total Guide Portions	My Total Portions
		Calibration			First Habit Foods					
Breakfast	🖐								7	
Mid-Morning Snack	🖐								7	
Lunch	🖐🖐								14	
Afternoon Snack	🖐								7	
Dinner	🖐🖐								14	
Evening Snack	🖐								7	
Extra Portions										

Circle or shade your hand portions for each meal.

Total [ ]

Check a box per each Social Food Meal

Social Foods	8 or Fewer/ Week									Total Social Foods

Drinks (8 oz.)	Way In Guide	Mon.	Tues.	Wed.	Thurs.	Fri.	Sat.	Sun.	Total Guide Drinks	My Total Drinks
Water & Non-Caloric Drinks	8-10/ Day								56-70	
Caloric Drinks	1/ Day Max								7	
Extra Caloric Drinks										

Move	Way In Guide	Mon.	Tues.	Wed.	Thurs.	Fri.	Sat.	Sun.	Total Guide Minutes	My Total Minutes
		Baseline Strength, Stamina & Consistency								
Resistance	3 Days 20 min.	Min.	Min.	Min.	Min.	Min.	Min.	Min.	60	
Cardio/ Walking	4 Days 20-30 min.	Min.	Min.	Min.	Min.	Min.	Min.	Min.	60	
Standing	7 Days 60 min.	Min.	Min.	Min.	Min.	Min.	Min.	Min.	420	

What Went Right? *I felt leanest, strongest and most energized after:*

Top Foods: _____

Top Workouts: _____

What's Not For Me? *I felt bloated, drained or low energy after:*

Foods/Workouts: _____

Habit Food Calculator

Habit Food Portions ÷ Total Food Portions

x 100 =

Habit Food % Goal = 80%

NOTES

SIX WEEK SHAPE-UP: WEEK TWO

THE BIG PICTURE

This is your first week of the total lifestyle in full force. Stick to Habit Foods on your roster for 80% of your meals and have Social Foods only 20% of the time (in 7-8 meals per week).

On top of solidifying your basic Habit food strategy and eating schedule, your other focus this week will be on the physical sensation of satisfaction when you eat. Food is energy. And so is body fat. To lose weight, we need to get less energy from our plates and more from our personal stores (fat). If we stop eating at *satisfied* rather than full, we easily accomplish this.

As you log meals on your Week Two LIFEtracker Page, note if you're getting all the colors of the rainbow between your Habit Foods and Social Foods. Don't stress about getting every color every day. Just look at your weekly big picture to evaluate how colorful (nutritious) is your Habit Food plan and make adjustments as necessary. Hint: I often use dinners to catch up on colors missed throughout the day. Hint hint: Lean heavily on dark greens and add a few berries and baby carrots to your afternoon or evening snacks if your go-to's on a particular week aren't exactly a carousel of color.

Your movement goal this week is to up your exercise game with an overall higher intensity workouts by increasing intensity with. For each exercise session, you must include 10 minutes of resistance work every day. The AND/life™ app has tons of options between classes and custom workouts to fulfill this requirement. Keep in mind that, when you're consistent, less is absolutely more – 20 mins of dedicated, strategic work is plenty when combined with the rest of this program's life activation elements.

That said, if you're feeling it and want to work out longer, you can. But do not overdo it by upping both your intensity and duration more than three days this week. And limit yourself to sessions that are no longer than 40 minutes or your hunger will shoot up. First and foremost, the #1 goal is still about getting your stomach calibrated.

FOOD

Satisfied v. Full: Stop eating when you feel satisfied, even if you haven't finished your portion. This practice will help you develop a more intuitive relationship with your body and teach you to eat more in line with your actual energy needs.

- Follow the normal eating schedule and portion guidelines.

- Eat 80% Habit Foods from your worksheet and allow yourself 20% Social Foods.

- Stop eating the moment you are satisfied, before you feel full.

- Plan a to-do for right after you eat so you don't linger. (Bonus: use your Life List!)

Drinks: Continue with Weight Loss Strategy – 8-10 8oz. non-caloric, beneficial beverages each day, plus no more than one 8 oz. caloric drink per day.

Plan: Look ahead to next week's three "Clean Slate" days and adjust your Habit Food roster accordingly by adding Best Habit Food options that are dairy- and grain-free for each meal and two of your snacks.

- Make "Clean Slate" versions of your favorite Go-To's by substituting non-dairy and gluten-free ingredients

- Check out ideas in Chapter 13 of the Appendix or find recipes on the AND/life app

EXERCISE

- Exercise for at least 20 mins each day including 10 mins of resistance work

- Do not exceed 40 mins for any workout

- Record your workout times and notes on your LIFEtracker page

STANDING

- Stand an extra 60 mins each day (total, minutes do not have to be consecutive).

- Add an extra 20 mins each day of being "up and about."

NOTES

_____

_____

_____

_____

_____

_____

_____

_____

_____

NOTES

_____

_____

_____

_____

_____

_____

_____

_____

_____

_____

_____

_____

_____

_____

_____

_____

LIFE*tracker*

WEEK 2

	Start Weight		End Weight		Change In Weight	Goal = 2lbs.

Habit Food Meals	Way In Portion Guide	Mon.	Tues.	Wed.	Thurs.	Fri.	Sat.	Sun.	Total Guide Portions	My Total Portions
		Satisfied vs. Full								
Breakfast									7	
Mid-Morning Snack									7	
Lunch									14	
Afternoon Snack									7	
Dinner									14	
Evening Snack									7	
Extra Portions										

Circle or shade your hand portions for each meal.

Total

Check a box per each Social Food Meal

Social Foods	8 or Fewer/ Week									Total Social Foods

Drinks (8 oz.)	Way In Guide	Mon.	Tues.	Wed.	Thurs.	Fri.	Sat.	Sun.	Total Guide Drinks	My Total Drinks
Water & Non-Caloric Drinks	8-10/ Day								56-70	
Caloric Drinks	1/ Day Max								7	
Extra Caloric Drinks										

Move	Way In Guide	Mon.	Tues.	Wed.	Thurs.	Fri.	Sat.	Sun.	Total Guide Minutes	My Total Minutes
		Increase Intensity: Daily Resistance Work								
Resistance	7 Days 10 min.	Min.	Min.	Min.	Min.	Min.	Min.	Min.	70	
Cardio/ Walking	7 Days 10-30 min.	Min.	Min.	Min.	Min.	Min.	Min.	Min.	70 Minimum	
Standing	7 Days 60 min.	Min.	Min.	Min.	Min.	Min.	Min.	Min.	420	

What Went Right? *I felt leanest, strongest and most energized after:*

Top Foods: _____

Top Workouts: _____

What's Not For Me? *I felt bloated, drained or low energy after:*

Foods/Workouts: _____

Habit Food Calculator

Habit Food Portions	÷	Total Food Portions

x 100 =

Habit Food % Goal = 80%

SIX WEEK SHAPE-UP: WEEK THREE

THE BIG PICTURE

For Week Three, the "Clean Slate" week, you have three goals:

1) ratchet your stomach down a little further

2) further rid your system of excess fluid (bloating)

3) solidify the baseline from which we'll discover the best foods for your body

This week we will clear your digestive system even more with three "Clean Slate Days" featuring only Best Habit Foods and no Social Foods or caloric drinks. The goal is to optimize your system for the rest of the program so when a meal makes you feel bloated or sluggish, you'll know the culprit right away. This is NOT an official allergy test. We are simply eliminating foods that most commonly present digestive challenges for a few days (grains and dairy), so we can slowly reintroduce them and reveal how they may be negatively impacting your digestion and/or creating demoralizing short-term weight fluctuations.

The information we gather will also help us create your Rapid Reset at the end of this program, so be sure to keep notes in your Week Three LIFEtracker Page. The Rapid Reset will be one of the most powerful tools in your toolbox to help you stay in charge of your weight - a secret weapon plan for anytime you feel not so great or absolutely need to feel lean ASAP (i.e. an event or beach vacation).

Don't worry if you feel overwhelmed by the idea of coming up with all Best Habit Foods for three days - I have included a Clean Slate Days sample menu and recipes in Chapter 13the appendix of this book.

After three days of "cleaning your digestive slate," you will return to your basic Habit Food strategy which includes Social Foods and caloric drinks, but with the reintroduction of grains and dairy slowly.

Exercise-wise, you'll continue to get your heart rate up for at least 20 consecutive minutes each day. On your Clean Slate days, keep in mind that you'll have less fuel for intense workouts. The goal for those days is simply about exercise *consistency* over intensity.

FOOD

Days 1-3: Clean Slate eating—Fast track your stomach calibration, flush water, reduce bloating, and clear your body of grains and dairy so that when you reintroduce these foods, you can see how your body reacts to them.

- Eat only Best Habit Foods.

- Follow the lowest levels of portions:

    · Breakfast—One Hand

    · Snack—One Hand (2-4 hours later)

    · Lunch—Two Hands (2-3 hours later)

    · Snack—One Hand (2 hours later)

    · Dinner—One and a Half Hands (2-3 hours later)

    · Post Dinner Snack—One Hand (2 hours later)

- Do not eat Social Foods.

- Do not drink caloric beverages aside from a splash of milk in your coffee.

Days 4-7: Learning About Grains—Return to your Habit Foods Strategy with only one serving of grains per day and still no dairy foods.

- Eat both Best and Limited Habit Foods.

- Stick to only one Social Food and one caloric drink per day.

- Return to the original hand-portioning guidelines of the lifestyle.

- Each day at one meal, test a one-hand portion of a single grain and keep an eye out for changes in how you feel over the rest of the day.

- Continue to avoid dairy products in both Habit and Social Foods.

- Continue with weight loss approach to caloric drinks – only one per day.

Plan:

- If you haven't already, add new recipe options from your Clean Slate days to your Habit Foods Worksheet for future reference.

- Schedule your success by continuing to alternate only 2-3 favorite Habit Food options for breakfasts, lunches and snack times each week.

- Even though we are constantly adding ideas to your Habit Foods Worksheet, change your current Go-To's only when you get bored —and try to only change one or two options per week so as not to be too disruptive to your schedule or add other variables while testing grains and dairy.

- Dinners may continue to be different most days. Again, totally fine.

EXERCISE

- For Clean Slate days (days 1-3), walk or do moderate cardio, 20-30 minutes each.

- For days 4-7, do 20-30 minutes total of any combination of exercise including 10 minutes of resistance work. You can find strength training, Pilates, or yoga classes on the AND/life™ app to get your resistance in.

STANDING

- Stand an extra 60 mins each day (total, minutes do not have to be consecutive).

- Include an extra 20 mins of casual movement each day.

LEARN

Grains

For some people, grains can be bloating, inflammatory, or take longer to digest. Are you one of these people? There's only one way to find out!

This week pay close attention to how you feel without grains and what changes after you reintroduce them. Do you feel more or less tired? Bloated? Some people may choose to move certain grains to the Social Foods category because they feel better without them. Some may not feel any difference at all. The only way to know which type of person you are is to experiment and figure out how you can feel your best. If you notice significant discomfort when reintroducing any particular grain, see a doctor for a true sensitivity or allergy test.

NOTES

_____

_____

_____

_____

_____

_____

LIFE *tracker*

WEEK 3

	Start Weight		End Weight		Change In Weight		Goal = 2lbs.

Habit Food Meals	Way In Portion Guide	Mon.	Tues.	Wed.	Thurs.	Fri.	Sat.	Sun.	Total Guide Portions	My Total Portions
			Clean Slate Days			Grain Test Sprint				
Breakfast									7	
Mid-Morning Snack									7	
Lunch									14	
Afternoon Snack									7	
Dinner									14	
Evening Snack									7	
Extra Portions										

Circle or shade your hand portions for each meal.

Total

Check a box per each Social Food Meal

Social Foods	4 or Fewer/ Week									Total Social Foods

Drinks (8 oz.)	Way In Guide	Mon.	Tues.	Wed.	Thurs.	Fri.	Sat.	Sun.	Total Guide Drinks	My Total Drinks
Water & Non-Caloric Drinks	8-10/ Day								56-70	
Caloric Drinks	4/ Week Max								4	
Extra Caloric Drinks										

Move	Way In Guide	Mon.	Tues.	Wed.	Thurs.	Fri.	Sat.	Sun.	Total Guide Minutes	My Total Minutes
			Days 1-3: Moderate Cardio	Days 4-7: Resistance Work						
Resistance	Days 4-7 10 min.	Min.	Min.	Min.	Min.	Min.	Min.	Min.	40	
Cardio/ Walking	7 Days 10-30 min.	Min.	Min.	Min.	Min.	Min.	Min.	Min.	70 Minimum	
Standing	7 Days 60 min.	Min.	Min.	Min.	Min.	Min.	Min.	Min.	420	

What Went Right? *I felt leanest, strongest and most energized after:*

Top Foods: _____

Top Workouts: _____

What's Not For Me? *I felt bloated, drained or low energy after:*

Foods/Workouts: _____

Habit Food Calculator

Habit Food Portions ÷ Total Food Portions

x 100 =

Habit Food % Goal = 80%

NOTES

SIX WEEK SHAPE-UP: WEEK FOUR

THE BIG PICTURE

This week, you have two objectives:

1. Discover how your body reacts to dairy products.

2. Leave a bite or two of food on your plate at every meal.

You will reintroduce dairy on the first day of the week this week. As with grains, it will be important to be sure to note how this any particular dairy foods affects your body on your Week Four LIFEtracker page. Since you are adding a potentially complicated food back into your rotation, in these first few days, stick with Habit Foods you know work for you rather than trying new ones. This will help make it stand out if you have a possible sensitivity to dairy you don't know about. Watch for obvious signs like bloating, gas or indigestion, and also later- or next-day puffiness in your face or hands or aching joints – signs of inflammation. On a more positive note, some people who think they have a dairy issue (not diagnosed by a doctor, just a feeling) sometimes learn they digest dairy fine as long as the portions are small.

Last week you listened to your stomach and made a commitment to stop eating when you were full. This week, we'll take it one step further by including a formal check: leave one or two bites. Even if you weren't raised with the "Clean Plate Club," seeing something unfinished is difficult for our human psychology psyche. By making a conscious effort to leave a bite or two on your plate at every meal, you'll desensitize yourself to the uncomfortable sight of a little left over, seeing the "task" of eating a meal not finished. This will help solidify the game-changing life habit of eating to the point of satisfied instead of full.

Leaving a little bite is especially important now, at the Week Four mark, when "portion creep" starts to happen. Once people get into an established roster of meals and have seen the scale moving consistently for a few weeks, they tend to get a bit overconfident and more lenient with how they eye-ball their portions: spoonful's of nut butter begin to overflow; the piece of chicken you choose gets a little bigger; the glass of wine you pour is a little more generous...

Remember, it's crucial that food portions stay in check so that you can have freedom with Social Foods. Also, this week we will start approaching caloric drinks from a lifestyle perspective – you will be allowed up to two per day. Proper food portions prevent calories you may drink from derailing your efforts.

This week for exercise, you will up the amount of resistance work you do, but not necessarily your total workout time. This will allow you to continue building baseline strength and stamina without increasing your hunger or affecting your new schedule before it becomes ingrained. Creating a consistent, manageable amount of time every day to get your heart rate up is one of the most life-changing aspects of this program. A physique that results from a strategy that can be maintained no matter what life throws at you is one you will get to keep.

FOOD

Calibration Double-Check: Leave one or two bites of your two-hand meals to mentally train yourself to stop seeing food as "unfinished business."

Dairy Products: If you eat dairy, begin to add it back into your schedule.

- Eat a one-hand portion of a dairy Habit Food on its own as a snack each day. Social Foods may contain dairy as well, keep to no more than one one-handed portion.

- Remember the Rule of Awesome: if it's not awesome, don't eat it! You—and your waistline—deserve better!

Drinks: Lifestyle Strategy – The Way In allows for up to two caloric drinks per day. But if your weight loss slows, caloric drinks will be the first place to make an adjustment for next week.

- Aim for 8-10 non-caloric, beneficial beverages (8 oz.) each day

- Up to 2 caloric drinks (8 oz.) per day

Plan: Add more new Habit Foods, including one breakfast, lunch, and two snacks that are only made of Best Habit Foods ingredients. Find three new dinner options that are from the Best group as well. If you're bored with some foods on your current roster, go ahead and switch them out. But try to not make too many changes or overcomplicate things.

EXERCISE

This week you will still focus on stamina and strength, but you will also increase your cardio capacity and metabolic "afterburn" with HIIT.

- 3 HIIT 10-20-minute workouts.

- 3 heavy resistance 10-20-minute workouts. Add 10-20 minutes moderate cardio to any workout. Make one day an active rest day – only walk for 20-60 minutes.

STANDING

- Stand an extra 90 mins each day (total, does not have to be consecutive).

- Include an extra 20 mins of casual, "up-and-about" movement each day.

LEARN

Dairy

Like grains, dairy is not "bad," but depending on your body, it may have many unfortunate side effects, like bloating, skin maladies, gastrointestinal trouble, fatigue, or inflammation. Pay close attention to how you feel this week as you reintroduce this food group back into your schedule. If you don't like the way your body reacts, make this a food you eat less of, or even cut it out of your rotation.

Your Fuel Needs

Are you still hungry or just bored? Are you haunted by the "Clean Plate Club" of years gone by? As you eat this week, really focus on your stomach as you near the end of each meal. Remember that your plate is not another project on your to-do list that must be finished. "Just a few bites" meal after meal, day after day, adds up to a whole lot of food. Strategize the habit of putting your fork down when you know your body doesn't need any more and you will begin to shed pounds and prevent adding unnecessary fuel to your system which will be stored as fat.

NOTES

_____

_____

_____

_____

_____

_____

LIFE*tracker*

WEEK 4

	Start Weight		End Weight		Change In Weight	Goal = 2lbs.

Habit Food Meals	Way In Portion Guide	Mon.	Tues.	Wed.	Thurs.	Fri.	Sat.	Sun.	Total Guide Portions	My Total Portions
		Leave 1-2 Bites & Dairy Test Sprint								
Breakfast									7	
Mid-Morning Snack									7	
Lunch									14	
Afternoon Snack									7	
Dinner									14	
Evening Snack									7	
Extra Portions										

Circle or shade your hand portions for each meal.

Total

Check a box per each Social Food Meal

Social Foods	8 or Fewer/ Week													Total Social Foods

Drinks (8 oz.)	Way In Guide	Mon.	Tues.	Wed.	Thurs.	Fri.	Sat.	Sun.	Total Guide Drinks	My Total Drinks
Water & Non-Caloric Drinks	8-10/ Day								56-70	
Caloric Drinks	2/ Day Max								14 Max	
Extra Caloric Drinks										

Move	Way In Guide	Mon.	Tues.	Wed.	Thurs.	Fri.	Sat.	Sun.	Total Guide Minutes	My Total Minutes
		Increase Intensity: HIIT Workouts								
HIIT	3 Days 10-20 min.	Min.	Min.	Min.	Min.	Min.	Min.	Min.	30 Minimum	
Med/Heavy Resistance	3 Days 10 min.	Min.	Min.	Min.	Min.	Min.	Min.	Min.	30	
Cardio/ Walking	7 Days 10-60 min.	Min.	Min.	Min.	Min.	Min.	Min.	Min.	70 Minimum	
Standing	7 Days 90 min.	Min.	Min.	Min.	Min.	Min.	Min.	Min.	630	

What Went Right? *I felt leanest, strongest and most energized after:*

Top Foods: _____

Top Workouts: _____

What's Not For Me? *I felt bloated, drained or low energy after:*

Foods/Workouts: _____

Habit Food Calculator

Habit Food Portions ÷ Total Food Portions

x 100 =

Habit Food % Goal = 80%

NOTES

SIX WEEK SHAPE-UP: WEEK FIVE

THE BIG PICTURE

The next two weeks are about cementing your new habits and strategies so that exercising 20 minutes each day, standing at least 90 and eating go-to foods you can easily make yourself 80% of the time become your way of life. Commit to showing up for yourself each and every day!

By now, your tastes have definitely adjusted to prefer cleaner, simpler foods, with less sugar and salt. For this reason, you might find those dishes you've been looking forward to having for your social meals are less appealing. Don't be disappointed that you no longer enjoy a whole bag of greasy potato chips. Embrace your new tastes, stop with just a few and be thrilled for proof that you are growing and changing for the better!

You will also perform another food "test sprint" this week to see how you react to fruit. Yes, fruit is good for humans. But no, not everyone processes it the same. You may benefit from eating it more strategically—and this is the week you'll find out!

Now that you have the "food thing" down, your body will start a slow and steady slimming process that won't let up unless you do. And since your new food "lifestyle" involves eating socially 7-8 times per week, there is no reason to let up, right? Your body should be starting to reveal all the gorgeous muscle you've been hiding under all those excess-energy-layers (aka flab).

This also means that now is the perfect time to get more strategic. Taking a brisk walk does count toward burning body fat and improving your cardio-vascular health. But walking alone won't get you the kind of arms you're dying to show off! To get the body of your dreams, you've got to continuously challenge yourself in new ways. We will start now by upping your weights 10-20% this week. Also, vary your exercise blend by trying different classes on the AND/life app or at your gym and watch how positively your body responds to the surprise!

FOOD

Your Regularly Scheduled Program—Plan out the foods you'll alternate for breakfasts, lunches, snacks and dinners, shop for them and include Social Foods up to one time per day (or go totally clean a couple days and save up some Socials for the weekend). Up to two caloric drinks are still allowed, but on days you're fine with less, definitely do that.

Fruit Test "Sprint": Get a sense of your body's ability to handle fructose by eating a one hand portion of a favorite individual fruit for one snack each day.

To Do:

- For your mid-morning snack, have a one hand portion of fruit with nothing else.

- Eat the fruit at least two hours after and two hours before any other foods.

- If you can, try a different fruit each day. (Berries can be combined.)

Plan: Add one more breakfast, lunch, dinner and two snack options to your Habit Foods worksheets.

EXERCISE

This week you will focus on further development of your physique.

- Encourage greater shape and definition in your muscles by upping your weights slightly (i.e. 3 lbs goes to 5; 5 lbs goes to 8; 10 lbs to 12 or 15... you get the idea).

- "Medium" resistance means a weight that is very challenging by 15-20 repetitions.

- "Heavy" resistance means a weight that makes only 10 repetitions of an exercise doable.

- Alternate resistance and bodyweight work this week: Do two 20 minute heavy weight workouts this week.

- Do three body-weight workouts (i.e. HIIT, Pilates, Yoga)Pilates or Yoga classes may be 20-60 minutes.

- HIIT workouts should be only 20-30 minutes.

- You may add up to 20 minutes of cardio to any workout, never to exceed 60 minutes. Do two moderate cardio days, 20-40 minutes.

STANDING

- Stand an extra 90 mins each day (total, minutes do not have to be consecutive).

- Include an extra 20 mins of casual movement each day.

LEARN

Fruit

Fruit is a key Best Habit Food because it provides serious nutritional benefits – vitamins, fiber, water, energy (and happiness – yum!). But we need to have a sense of how much fructose our own individual body can handle at one time and throughout the day. For most of my clients, 1-2 servings of fruit per day (with a few hours in between) allows them to lose excess body fat while adding valuable nutrition to their everyday eating plan.

This week, take note of how you feel after you eat fruit. Do you feel more energetic? Do you feel quickly "hungry" for something else? Do you feel bloated and puffy, or do you feel light and lean? Note any digestive discomfort you feel within the next few hours. If a fruit seems to bother you, maybe try it again with only half the amount and paired with a protein or fat.

By the end of this week, you'll know if fruit may be keeping you from feeling your best, also if certain ones seem better than others. There are so many fantastic fruits, so keep experimenting as you progress beyond the program in this book. And even if you notice no issues digesting fruit, maybe stick to one-hand servings as a general rule since our bodies are so inefficient at deriving energy from fructose.

NOTES

LIFE tracker

WEEK 5

	Start Weight		End Weight		Change In Weight	Goal = 2lbs.

Habit Food Meals	Way In Portion Guide	Mon.	Tues.	Wed.	Thurs.	Fri.	Sat.	Sun.	Total Guide Portions	My Total Portions
					Fruit Test Sprint					
Breakfast									7	
Mid-Morning Snack									7	
Lunch									14	
Afternoon Snack									7	
Dinner									14	
Evening Snack									7	
Extra Portions										

Circle or shade your hand portions for each meal.

Total

Check a box per each Social Food Meal

Social Foods	8 or Fewer/ Week									Total Social Foods

Drinks (8 oz.)	Way In Guide	Mon.	Tues.	Wed.	Thurs.	Fri.	Sat.	Sun.	Total Guide Drinks	My Total Drinks
Water & Non-Caloric Drinks	8-10/ Day								56-70	
Caloric Drinks	2/ Day Max								14 Max	
Extra Caloric Drinks										

Move	Way In Guide	Mon.	Tues.	Wed.	Thurs.	Fri.	Sat.	Sun.	Total Guide Minutes	My Total Minutes
				Vary Exercise Blend	Increase Resistance & Workout Duration					
Pilates or Yoga	2 Days 20-60 min.	Min.	Min.	Min.	Min.	Min.	Min.	Min.	40 Minimum	
Med/Heavy Resistance	3 Days 20 min.	Min.	Min.	Min.	Min.	Min.	Min.	Min.	60	
Cardio/ Walking	7 Days 20-40 min.	Min.	Min.	Min.	Min.	Min.	Min.	Min.	140 Minimum	
Standing	7 Days 90 min.	Min.	Min.	Min.	Min.	Min.	Min.	Min.	630	

What Went Right? *I felt leanest, strongest and most energized after:*

Top Foods: _____

Top Workouts: _____

What's Not For Me? *I felt bloated, drained or low energy after:*

Foods/Workouts: _____

Habit Food Calculator

Habit Food Portions ÷ Total Food Portions

x 100 =

Habit Food % Goal = 80%

NOTES

SIX WEEK SHAPE-UP: WEEK SIX

THE BIG PICTURE

This week, your last official program week, you'll be converting the "plan" into a way of life.

Continue discerning when you're <u>satisfied</u> at each meal – which is sometimes before you finish your one/two hand portion. If you're having a "hungry day" and honestly need a few more bites than you portioned yourself, eat them. You know yourself now, so honor what your body is telling you. With that said, check in on yourself each meal and be sure. If the scale starts going up and not coming down again, you're doing the "slow creep" with your portions.

A few times when you eat out or on the run this week, practice adjusting restaurant offerings to fit Habit Food parameters—the cleanest ingredients and the simplest preparation. The objective is to prove to yourself that you always have the power to stick to your personal plan and enjoy yourself just as much. And when the Rule of Awesome applies and you choose the decadent cake, you can do so with no more guilt and no more crazy "diet" derailments. Meals for you are now simply about strategic choices that create room to allow extraordinary food to be a key part of your life.

Regarding exercise, this last week we will make a final strength and stamina push before you move beyond this program and into "lifestyle mode." This week only, blend exercise types to create longer workouts for total workouts of 30-60 minutes.

After this, staying consistent with at least 20 minutes per day, including at least three 20-minute resistance workouts per week, will be plenty to keep you headed toward your best self – which may be even better than what you thought possible!

You will also spend time looking back on your journey. Using your LIFEtracker pages, you will fill out your progress analysis immediately following this chapter. This tool will help you recap which foods and activities worked best for you and determine your "personal fitness formula."

Always remember as you continue with your Habit Food Strategy beyond these six weeks that the scale will never stay in the same place. In fact, it will probably go up and down a bit every day. Overall, however, you will see a downward trend until you get to your goal. As you live this lifestyle a while and prove to yourself a few times that you now know how your body works and what to do when you see the scale go up a bit, those fluctuations will stop having an emotional impact on you. And that's when you will be truly free to enjoy food – and your life in some very important ways – a whole lot more!

FOOD

Put It All Together.

To Do:

- Continue alternating your favorite Habit Foods and sticking to portion and schedule guidelines.

- For every meal at a restaurant this week, make a point to choose options that fit Habit Foods guidelines or modify available options to make them fit.

Plan: Continue to expand your personal Habit Foods library by adding one new breakfast, lunch, and dinner and two more snacks. You should finish with 6 go-to's for breakfast and lunch, 10 dinner ideas and 12 snack options.

EXERCISE

- Do three 30-60 min workouts with at least 20 min resistance work with med-heavy weights plus walking/cardio.

- Do four 30-60 min workouts with at least 20 min HIIT or lengthening work (yoga or Pilates) plus walking/cardio.

- Do not do more than 3 workouts that are longer than 45 mins.

STANDING

- Stand an extra 90 mins each day (total, minutes do not have to be consecutive).

- Include an extra 20 mins of casual movement each day.

LEARN

Look Back to Move Forward

At the end of this week, complete your progress analysis to unlock your "personal fitness formula." Using your LIFEtracker Pages from the previous six weeks, fill out your Fitness Lifestyle and Rapid Reset worksheets on pages 130 and 131. These formulas will be your personal roadmap toward your fitness goals beyond the Six Week Shape-Up.

NOTES

_____

_____

_____

_____

NOTES

WEEK 6

| Start Weight | | End Weight | | Change In Weight | | Goal = 2lbs. |

Habit Food Meals	Way In Portion Guide	Mon.	Tues.	Wed.	Thurs.	Fri.	Sat.	Sun.	Total Guide Portions	My Total Portions
		Satisfied vs. Full & Dining Out: Habit Food Modifications								
Breakfast	🖐								7	
Mid-Morning Snack	🖐								7	
Lunch	🖐🖐								14	
Afternoon Snack	🖐								7	
Dinner	🖐🖐								14	
Evening Snack	🖐								7	
Extra Portions										

Circle or shade your hand portions for each meal.

| | | | | | | | | | | Total |

Check a box per each Social Food Meal

| Social Foods | 8 or Fewer/ Week | | | | | | | | | Total Social Foods |

Drinks (8 oz.)	Way In Guide	Mon.	Tues.	Wed.	Thurs.	Fri.	Sat.	Sun.	Total Guide Drinks	My Total Drinks
Water & Non-Caloric Drinks	8-10/ Day								56-70	
Caloric Drinks	2/ Day Max								14 Max	
Extra Caloric Drinks										

Move	Way In Guide	Mon.	Tues.	Wed.	Thurs.	Fri.	Sat.	Sun.	Total Guide Minutes	My Total Minutes
		Final Push: Increased Duration & Varied Exercise Blend								
HIIT, Pilates or Yoga + Cardio	4 Days 30-60 min.	Min.	Min.	Min.	Min.	Min.	Min.	Min.	100 Minimum	
Med/Heavy Resistance + Cardio	3 Days 30-60 min.	Min.	Min.	Min.	Min.	Min.	Min.	Min.	60 Minimum	

What Went Right? *I felt leanest, strongest and most energized after:*

Top Foods: _____

Top Workouts: _____

What's Not For Me? *I felt bloated, drained or low energy after:*

Foods/Workouts: _____

Habit Food Calculator

| Habit Food Portions | ÷ | Total Food Portions |

x 100 =

| Habit Food % Goal = 80% |

FITNESS LIFESTYLE *formula*

You're Almost There!

You've made a huge change in your life, and you're starting to see the benefits. It's time to add up what has worked best for you to find your "personal fitness formula"—your surefire lifestyle strategy for getting in shape, staying in shape, and loving your life along the way. Your personal Way In!

Using your LIFE*tracker* notes as a guide, circle the weeks you lost at least one pound. For those weeks only, answer the following questions: *(Check all boxes that apply.)*

Weeks	1	2	3	4	5	6
Which weeks did you feel your leanest?	Leanest	Leanest	Leanest	Leanest	Leanest	Leanest
Which weeks did you feel your strongest?	Strongest	Strongest	Strongest	Strongest	Strongest	Strongest
Which weeks did you feel the most energetic?	Energetic	Energetic	Energetic	Energetic	Energetic	Energetic

Refer to your LIFE*tracker* notes from the top 3 weeks above *(the ones with the most checked boxes)* to answer the following questions: *(Check all boxes that apply.)*

Workouts	HIIT	Pilates / Yoga	Resistance / Weights	Walking / Cardio
Which workouts were the easiest to fit into your schedule?	Fit Schedule	Fit Schedule	Fit Schedule	Fit Schedule
Which workouts left you feeling powerful and uplifted?	Powerful & Uplifted	Powerful & Uplifted	Powerful & Uplifted	Powerful & Uplifted
Which workouts did you find pure fun?	Pure Fun	Pure Fun	Pure Fun	Pure Fun

Progress Strategy Calculator

Social Meals	Top Week 1	+ Top Week 2	+ Top Week 3	= Total	÷ 3 =	Avg. Social Meals/Wk
Caloric Drinks	Top Week 1	+ Top Week 2	+ Top Week 3	= Total	÷ 3 =	Avg. Social Meals/Wk

Fitness Lifestyle Formula

Congratulations! You've now discovered your Fitness Lifestyle Formula:

- Follow food schedule and portion guidelines.
- Lean on Habit Foods from the top 3 weeks above.
- Allow yourself up to _____ Social Meals each week.
- Allow yourself up to _____ Caloric Drinks each week.
- Get your heart rate up at least 20 min/day, alternating _____ *(Top Workout 1)* and _____ *(Top Workout 2)* 4-5 times each week.
- Stand at least 90 minutes each day.

RAPID RESET *formula*

FOOD STRATEGY

Using your LIFE*tracker* notes from the top 2 weeks you lost the most weight, list your favorite meal of each day: *(Write in the boxes below.)*

Breakfast	Mid-Morning Snacks	Lunch	Afternoon Snacks	Dinner	Evening Snacks

WORKOUT STRATEGY

Using your LIFE*tracker* notes from the top 2 weeks you lost the most weight, list your favorite 3 workouts: *(Write in the boxes below.)*

Favorite Workout 1	Favorite Workout 2	Favorite Workout 3

Rapid Reset Formula

Woo hoo! You've now created your Rapid Reset for times when you need a kickstart or a come-back. Follow these food and excercise choices for 3-7 days when you need a fast-track to feeling your leanest, strongest and most energetic.

- Eat only the Habit Food meal options listed above, following usual schedule and portion guidelines.
- Drink only non-caloric beverages.
- Get your heart rate up for at least 20 minutes each day, choosing from amongst the 3 workouts listed above.
- Stand at least 90 minutes each day.

12

CHEAT SHEETS

SAMPLE HABIT FOOD MEALS

Here are some quick Habit Food recipe ideas from my AND/life™ app. Please don't make every meal a big deal or this will become a "diet" you can't maintain. As you'll see, many of my "recipes" are hardly that (i.e., the culinary masterpiece of a snack I have named: "Apple and Cheese.")

The app makes Habit Food planning even easier by sorting through hundreds of Habit Food recipes to suggest options. A weekly menu based on your personal goals and ingredients you choose, while keeping in mind allergies and preferences (i.e., vegetarian, vegan, no red meat, etc.). You can also add recipes from the library that sound good to you into your rotation. Check it out!

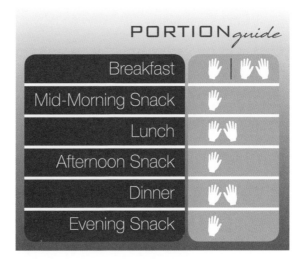

Breakfast (One-Hand or Two Hand Portions)

- 2 Nut Butter Sandwich (one half)

- Make-Ahead Mini Crustless Quiche Egg Frittatas

- Birchermeusli (Swiss-style yogurt with oats, nuts and fruit)

- Yogurt (full fat) with Fresh Fruit

- Melon with Cottage Cheese (full fat) and 1 TBSP Sunflower or Chia Seeds

- Appwiches (Apple/Nut Butter Sandwiches)

- Egg & Avocado Sweet Potato Toast

- Veggie Omelet in a Mug

- Yogurt (full fat) with Fresh Fruit

- Egg Whites with Avocado OR Shredded Cheese

- High Quality Bar (Requires refrigeration, low or no grains, sugar <20g)

Morning Snack (One-Hand Portions)

- Apple and Cheese

- Fruit plus 10 Almonds or Walnuts

- Nut Butter Sandwich (one half)

- Yogurt & Chia Seeds (full fat, no fruit flavors or syrup)

- 1-2 Hard-Boiled Eggs (eat only one yolk); season with pepper or hot sauce

- Any breakfast item

Lunch (Two-Hand Portions)

- Turkey & Avocado Romaine Roll-Ups
- Chicken, Tuna or Egg Salad over Spinach Mixed Greens
- PB&J Smoothie
- Open-Faced Sandwich with Veggies – Turkey, Chicken, Hummus, etc.
- Greek Zoodles
- Tuna Nicoise Wrap
- Quinoa Black Bean Salad
- Vegetable Mini Tacos
- Turkey Chili with Avocado and Field Greens
- Habit Food Dinner Leftovers

Afternoon Snack (One-Hand Portions)

- Turkey Meatballs in Spicy Tomato Sauce
- One-Hand Dinner Protein
- 70% Dark Chocolate & Peanut (1-2 oz.)
- ½ Nut Butter Sandwich
- 2 Hard-Boiled Eggs (eat only one or two yolks per day)
- A Cappuccino (whole milk or, if dairy-free, choose a plant milk with protein)
- Zucchini Avocado Hummus with Raw Veggies
- Hemp or Oat Milk Matcha Latte
- Two Spoons: Sunflower Seed Butter Spoonful & Pure Fruit Spread Spoonful
- Salad Greens with 1 TBSP Homemade Olive-Oil Based Dressing
- Thai Tofu Vegetable Curry Soup
- Any breakfast or morning snack
- Habit Food Dinner Leftovers

Dinner (Two-Hand Portions)

- Fast Turkey Chili and Baby Greens

- Single-Pan Roast Chicken and Broccoli

- Pork Chops and Market Vegetables

- Grilled Steak and Sautéed Brussels Sprouts with Walnuts

- Chicken Fajita Bowl over Brown Rice or Sautéed Spinach with Home-made Guacamole

- Meatballs (turkey or lean ground beef) over Pasta* with Romaine Salad

- Pasta* Primavera with Sautéed Shrimp or Leftover Roast Chicken

- Veggie Lasagna*

- Slow-Cooker Chicken Thighs over Cauliflower "Rice" with Sautéed Asparagus Spears

- Homemade Veggie Burgers with Kale Chips

- Lettuce-wrapped Turkey Cheeseburgers with Roasted Sweet Potato "Chips"

- Curried Red Lentil Soup with Lemony Spinach Salad

- Skirt Steak with Chimichurri Sauce and Edie's Love Salad Arugula/Heart of Palm/Walnut salad

- Eggplant Rollatini with "Simpler Caesar" Salad

- Organic/All-Natural Chicken Sausage, White Bean and Kale Soup

- Garlic Shrimp over Sautéed Spinach

Nighttime Snack (One-Hand Portions)

- Leftover Dinner (or just more of the veggies)

- Roasted Veggies

- 70% Dark Chocolate (1-2 oz.)

- Grapefruit, Melon or Berries

- Roasted Cauliflower Hummus with Cucumbers

- Clean Slate Soup

- Cheese Slice-Wrapped Roast Turkey

- Apple Slices

- Baby Carrots

To count as a Habit Food, pasta must be whole-grain or bean-based. If using regular white pasta, consider it a Social Meal.

Great "Green" Vegetables: Fibrous, non-starchy vegetable ideas for "lean and green" meals

Artichoke & Artichoke hearts (watch sodium if canned or jarred)

Asparagus

Baby corn (watch sodium if canned or jarred)

Bamboo shoots

Beans (green, wax, Italian, yard long)

Bean sprouts

Beets

Brussels sprouts

Broccoli

Cabbage (green, red, bok choy, Chinese)

Carrots

Cauliflower

Celery

Coleslaw (packaged without dressing – you make your own)

Cucumber

Daikon radish

Eggplant

Greens (collard, kale, mustard, turnip, Swiss chard, rainbow chard)

Hearts of palm

Jicama

Mushrooms

Okra

Onions, Leeks

Pea pods

Peppers

Radishes

Salad greens (i.e., baby greens, romaine, arugula, radicchio, endive, escarole, watercress)

Spinach

Sprouts

Squash (i.e., summer, crookneck, spaghetti, zucchini)

Sugar snap peas

Tomato

Turnips

Water chestnuts

BENEFICIAL FATS CHEAT SHEET

Plant-Based Beneficial Fats:

Extra Virgin Olive Oil

Coconut/Coconut Oil

Chia Seeds

Avocados

Walnuts

Almonds

Macadamia nuts

Pecans

Pistachios

Flax seeds (ground or oil – your body cannot digest whole flax seeds)

Pumpkin Seeds

Hemp Seeds

Animal-Based Beneficial Fat:

Fatty Fish - salmon

Yogurt (Full Fat)

Dark Chocolate

Cheese

Eggs (Whole)

Grass Fed Meats[1] (in limited amounts) (*What?* Yes.)

Grass Fed Butter (in limited amounts)

---

1 Yes, unrefined animal fats do raise LDL (low density lipoprotein) cholesterol – commonly known as "the bad kind." But that is not the whole story as there are *two kinds* of LDLs - a light, fluffy kind that does no harm and the small, hard particle kind that creates plaque build-up in your arteries. Animal fats raise the floaty kind of LDL, not the artery-clogging kind. But they also raise HDL (high density lipoprotein) - the "good" kind that lowers your risk of heart disease. So when you hear that "butter is OK" or wonder about me saying people who do dairy should drink whole milk, that's why. Let sodium be your check and balance on meats as Limited Habit Foods (twice per week). Those that are high in sodium are also highly processed (i.e., cured meats, sausage, bacon, turkey bacon, etc.) and don't qualify as Habit Foods at all.

High Heat Cooking Oils – 400°F and above

Grapeseed Oil

Avocado Oil

Walnut Oil

Coconut Oil (refined)

Oils to Avoid (foods cooked with these are Social Foods)

Soybean Oil

Canola Oil

Corn Oil

Cottonseed Oil

Sunflower Oil

Peanut Oil

Sesame Oil

"CLEAN SLATE" SAMPLE MEAL PLAN

Clean Slate days are a fast-lane way to optimize your system so you'll be working with a "clean slate" when you test grains, dairy and fructose during the Six Week Shape-Up. Clean Slate days have the added benefit of ratcheting your stomach size down a peg, eliminating inflammation, and helping change your tastes away from sugar and salt.

During Clean Slate, eat only "Best" Habit Foods, eliminating grains and dairy, and avoid all caloric beverages (not counting a splash of non-dairy milk in your morning coffee).

Each day choose one of the given options for each mealtime:

Breakfast: One hand

Clean Slate Superfood Bowl (one cup = one hand)

Clean Slate "Cup-let"

Hidden Greens Smoothie

Mid-morning: (2-4 hrs later) One hand

1 Hard-Boiled Egg

2 Apple Sandwiches

⅛ C Nuts

Lunch: (2-3 hrs later) Two hand

> Hot: Chicken/Green Veg Combo with Hot Sauce
>
> Cold: Turkey Lettuce Wraps with Peppers, Avocado, Squeeze of Lemon
>
> Veg: Hummus Open-Faced Zliders

Afternoon: (2 hrs later) One-hand

> 1 C Roasted Veggies: Broccoli or Brussels Sprouts
>   (use grapeseed, walnut or avocado oil) & 1/8 Cup nuts
>
> 1 C Clean Slate Soup
>
> 1 C Leftover Lunch or Dinner

Dinner: (2-3 hrs later) One and a half hand:

> Hot: Fish or Chicken with Spinach (sautéed in garlic
>   or raw as a salad with red wine vinegar)
>
> Hot: Clean Slate Soup
>
> Cold: Zoodles with Pesto and Chicken, Shrimp or Salmon

Nighttime: (2-4 hrs later) One-hand (pick any two)

> 1 TBSP Nut Butter (a spoonful)
>
> 1 C Spaghetti Squash Checca
>
> 1 C Baby Carrots with Zucchini/Avocado Hummus
>
> 1 Whole Grapefruit

Optional Extra (1 hr later)

> two or three bites of any Best Habit Food

CLEAN SLATE RECIPES

Clean Slate "Cup-let"

This one-minute omelet delivers quality protein, beneficial fats and a burst of vitamins and fiber from best veggies – all neat, tidy and portable in a mug.

1 large egg (or two egg whites if you can't do yolk)

¼ C "Best" Habit Food veggies, i.e., broccoli, kale, asparagus, red peppers

¼ avocado

Beat an egg with a fork in a coffee cup, drop in your veggies and microwave for about a minute, more or less depending on your microwave. Of course, you can also just do this in a nonstick pan sprayed with a little olive oil.

BTW, when you're not doing a Clean Slate Reset (which is no-grain/no-dairy to fight inflammation), feel free to try substituting 1 TBSP of whole milk shredded cheese when avocado isn't available – that's what I do!

Makes a single "one-hand" serving.

Clean Slate Superfood Bowl

Super-nutritious, this is one of my favorite "make-to-take" recipes for breakfast or a snack!

¾ C dairy-free vanilla yogurt

1 TBSP chopped walnuts, almonds, chia seeds OR nut butter

10 blueberries and/or 2 sliced strawberries

Swirl the nuts, seeds or nut butter into the yogurt and top with berries. Makes a single "one-hand" meal. For make-ahead servings, follow the same instructions and divide ingredients amongst five reusable 8oz containers using:

32oz yogurt

½ C nuts/seeds/nut butter

1 C blueberries/strawberries

Enjoy!

Hidden Greens Smoothie

Not too sweet, this smoothie has just the right amount of everything you need for a great breakfast, lunch or snack.

1 C hemp, oat or nut-based milk

¾ C frozen banana chunks

½ C blueberries and/or strawberries

1 Handful fresh spinach or kale

1 TBSP nut butter

1 TBSP local or 10+ Manuka honey (optional)

1 C ice (or more, if desired)

Blend all on high speed until well-incorporated, adding ice if desired.

This recipe equals a two-hand portion. Divide into two "one-hand" servings if you prefer. If you save some for later, the smoothie may lose some of its vibrant color. No worries – it'll still be delicious and nutritious!

Apple Sandwiches

Another great on-the-go breakfast or snack, apple sandwiches are packed with nutrition, fiber and that all-important "Yum!" factor.

1 Apple

1 ½ TBSP nut butter

Stand the apple on a cutting board and slice down one side three times. Give the apple a 1/3 turn and make three more slices. Turn and repeat one final time to finish the apple. You will end up with 6 "sandwich" slices and three end pieces (to snack on right now).

Fill each pair of sandwich slices with a generous teaspoon of nut butter. (Be sure to measure this the first time so you can see what a heaping teaspoon looks like on an apple slice. From then on, you'll be able to eyeball it pretty well.) Enjoy!

Warmed Checca Sauce

All the freshness and bite of a traditional Checca (which is basically chopped, seasoned, raw tomatoes), but with a little love from the stove for people like me who are: 1) saddened by tomato sauce without the "sauce," and 2) can't do raw garlic.

2 C fresh tomatoes (Roma or hothouse), diced small

2 cloves fresh garlic, rough chopped

1 TBSP extra-virgin olive or grapeseed oil

Pinch salt & pepper to taste

Warm oil over medium heat and then add garlic, heating just until it becomes fragrant – about one minute. Add the tomatoes and seasonings and cook down just slightly, covered, for no more than 5 minutes.

Serve over a lean protein and steamed spaghetti squash, zoodles (zucchini noodles) or a combination of sauteed veggies. Garnish with 2 TBSP torn basil.

Makes two "two-hand" servings.

Clean Slate Soup

Featuring high quality protein, fiber and nearly every color in the rainbow, you can't beat this soup for lunch, dinner or a snack during Clean Slate days – or any days, for that matter. Add water and adjust seasonings again the next day if your veggies soak up the broth. Considering a "two-hand" serving to equal about two cups, this recipe makes approximately 8-10 servings.

1 TBSP extra-virgin olive or grapeseed oil

1 small onion, diced

2 cloves fresh garlic, rough chopped

½ C sliced carrots

½ C sliced celery

1 C sliced green cabbage

1 28 oz can diced tomatoes (no salt if possible)

1 C garbanzo or kidney beans

8 cups (64 oz) Low-Sodium Bone, Chicken or Veggie Broth

Splash apple cider vinegar

1 tsp salt if desired and pepper to taste

1 TBSP Italian parsley (optional)

Warm the oil on med heat and brown the onion for about 5 mins, chopping other vegetables as you go. Add the garlic for one minute and then add carrots, celery, green cabbage and tomatoes as soon as each are ready. Rinse the beans well and then add, along with broth.

Bring to boil, then reduce heat. Add a splash of vinegar, salt if using and pepper. Partially cover and continue simmering on med-low heat for at least 30 minutes more.

Garnish with Italian parsley for a burst of nutrition and brightness. A splash of all-natural hot sauce is also a great way to make this simple soup sing!

Hummus Open-Faced Zliders

Crunch time! Satisfying, real-food munchies can make all the difference in getting you to your goals and keeping you there.

1 small zucchini

½ C hummus

1 red or yellow bell pepper or Roma tomato, sliced

Pinch of sea salt, if desired

Cracked pepper or hot sauce, to taste

Slice the zucchini lengthwise into four equal strips and then cut in half to make 8 pieces. Spread 1 TBSP hummus on each piece of zucchini, add pepper or tomato and seasoning. Enjoy!

13

A FINAL THOUGHT

HEY! LOOK AT YOU! You've made it through the program (or maybe you've skipped ahead and you're reading this before you start). Whichever, along the way, you've learned five principles that will guide your new healthy, abundant lifestyle. These tools are precisely what keeps this journey from being a diet that ends, and rather a foundation from which to live fully, richly and capably. The can-do mentality and commitment to yourself that it has taken for you to get to this page will serve you well, not only as you continue honing your new fitness lifestyle, but with any goals you set for yourself in life.

Physical strength builds mental strength and vice versa. Confidence about your "outside" opens you up, allowing you to share more of your "inside." And not to get all "kumbaya," but the skills, abilities and perspectives that we all hide for fear of being judged, are exactly the things that add valuable color, skills, perspective and heart to the world we all share. When you feel good about yourself, you put your best foot forward and that's a win for everyone. There's nothing selfish or narcissistic about this fitness journey you're on. Indeed, it's an act of generosity to set yourself up to be able to give your best.

Throughout the past six weeks, you've practiced **personal authenticity** by exploring your own personal path and breaking out of the expectations and standards set for you by others – or that you've set for yourself by comparing yourself to others. Start applying this standard to your life beyond food and exercise and watch doors to amazing opportunities swing wide open for you, while ones that suck your time and energy gently close.

You've also learned to **strategize your habits**, making sure that the best decisions you could make on your fitness journey are also the ones that are easiest and most natural. This goes for your life as a whole as well – the more no-brainers in your day, the fewer overall decisions, eliminating stress and creating time for more valuable things.

You've lived the **Rule of Awesome**, eating and drinking and doing the things that make you happiest—and not feeling guilty! And this doesn't just apply to calories in a day, but also time and money. Being discerning about how you spend your valuable resources makes taking your life up to the next level something you can afford. Pure enjoyment becomes plentiful without breaking your budget - calorically, time-wise or financially.

You've embraced **oppositional stability**, becoming flexible in order to roll with the challenges of your fitness journey, both physically and mentally. Embrace this concept – it's super effective far beyond the world of wellness and the less emotional stress you have, the better your body functions. The next time someone disagrees with you, try turning yourself around to see and understand their point of view first before responding. By the time you turn back, your perspective will be shifted just enough to put you on solid ground toward solutions rather than getting into a knock-down drag out where no one is left standing.

And all of these strategies have created time, strength and confidence to **allow in the extraordinary**: an amazing new version of yourself is beginning to take shape! Just as you have allowed this program to fruitfully detour you from your same old routine, keep your heart and mind open to other worthy risks or leaps of faith. Life offers all sorts of unexpected wonders and seemingly impossible opportunities. Some of life's greatest joys are found by simply being open to possibility and then, when they are offered, having the confidence to say YES.

Now, you absolutely will fail to live up to your best intentions at times. We all do. You will go to a buffet and eat all the cheese (and probably feel terrible afterward) or skip a week of the fitness classes you love. It's OK. You have a restart plan that can get you back to feeling your best quickly and a set of effective habits to ground yourself in from there. And you can move every single day—even if it's just a 20-minute walk. And you have a solid foundation of principles to call upon whenever you need a boost and to keep your overall life trajectory upward.

I'm so proud of you! I hope you are proud of you as well. Keep going. Keep showing up for yourself. And remember: There's no deadline for living your best life.

Your best life always starts right now.

ABOUT THE AUTHOR

ANDREA MARCELLUS is the Founder and CEO of her namesake lifestyle brand with a mission to help busy, driven people maximize their lives. A fitness expert and life strategist, Andrea has guided clients in New York and Los Angeles for 25 years. Over the past decade, Andrea honed and codified her unique, real-world fitness lifestyle into "5 Life Strategies," a learnable, actionable set of principles she uses to help her clients ramp up *every* area of their lives. These principles have become the foundation underpinning her company.

The Way In is the powerful intersection of Andrea's permission-based method to shaping up and her 5 Life Strategies. To make her mentality-boosting approach to fitness accessible anywhere and anytime, Andrea created *AND/life™*, the ultra-customizable app which serves as a companion to *The Way In*.

Andrea is an American Council on Exercise Certified Personal Trainer and received her Advanced Pilates Certification from IPC, Ivon Dahl. She holds numerous certifications including original Johnny G. Spinning, TRX, Cross-Core Training, Aerobics and Fitness Association of America (AFAA) Step and Group Fitness; RIPP Training, and has completed comprehensive continuing education in the field of nutrition.

An NYU graduate and screenwriter as well, Andrea's comedic feature film, *A Nice Girl Like You,* starring Lucy Hale, is slated for release in 2019.

Andrea lives in Los Angeles with her family and a menagerie of pets, including a bearded dragon.

APPENDIX

AS MUCH AS I'D LOVE FOR YOU TO CARRY THIS BOOK with you everywhere for six weeks while you do the Shape-Up, I recognize that this 1) may not be physically possible and 2) may be socially awkward. In the interest of your success, both with this program and with your social life, please enjoy quick reference pages of *The Way In* principles and extra copies of the worksheets found in this book.

THE 5 LIFE *strategies*

PRACTICE PERSONAL AUTHENTICITY

STRATEGIZE HABITS

LIVE THE RULE OF AWESOME

DEVELOP OPPOSITIONAL STABILITY

ALLOW IN THE EXTRAORDINARY

THE WAY IN LIFESTYLE:
DAILY GOALS AT A GLANCE

Food: schedule, portions, 80% Habit Foods

Hydration: 80% non-caloric drinks each week,
at least 8-10 glasses each day

Exercise: 20 minutes per day

Standing: 60 minutes per day to start working
your way up to at least 90 minutes

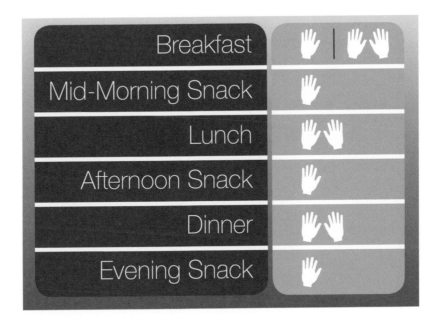

Breakfast	
Mid-Morning Snack	
Lunch	
Afternoon Snack	
Dinner	
Evening Snack	

BEST HABIT *foods*

Best Habit Foods
Energy With Optimal Nutritional Value

Non-Starchy Vegetables *(fresh or frozen)* • Fruits *(fresh or frozen)* • Lean Proteins
Beans • High Omega-3 Fish • Beneficial Fats • Nuts • Eggs

Limited Habit Foods
Energy With High Nutritional Value,
But Limit To Two Servings Or Less Each Day

Starchy Vegetables • Dairy & Cheese • Whole Grains • Honey and Pure Maple Syrup
Nut or Plant-Based Milks • All-Natural Dark Chocolate
High Quality Bars and Protein Powders • Red Meat *(2 per week)*

Preferred Social Foods
Energy With Some Nutritional Value And Some Detrimental Factors

Organic Dairy Products with Added Sugar • High Quality Bread & Pasta
Organic/All-Natural Packaged Foods • Juice, Wine

Low-Value Social Foods
Energy With Low Nutritional Value And A High Level Of Detrimental Factors

Sausage & Cured Meats • Packaged Foods with Chemical Preservatives • Non-Beneficial Fats
Fried Foods • Bleached Foods *(i.e., foods made with white flour)* • Canned Foods High In Sodium
High Fructose Foods Including Syrups, Nectars & Dried Fruits • Hard Alcohol